HEALTH EDUCATION

HEALTH EDUCATION

project of   Joint Committee on Health Problems in Education
of the National Education Association and the
American Medical Association

author   Robert D. Russell, Ed.D.
Professor of Health Education
Southern Illinois University

**medical
consultant**   Charles H. McMullen, M.D.
Loudonville, Ohio

Sixth Edition   Completely Rewritten, 1975

published by   National Education Association
1201 16th Street, N.W.
Washington, D.C. 20036

by NEA-AMA

other books   Healthful School Environment
School Health Services

NEA Order Department
Academic Building
order from   Saw Mill Road
West Haven, Connecticut 06516

American Medical Association
535 North Dearborn Street
Chicago, Illinois 60610

Library of Congress Cataloging in Publication Data

Russell, Robert D. 1926-
*   Health education.*

*   Includes bibliographical references.*
*   1. Health education. I. Joint Committee on Health*
Problems in Education. II. Title. [DNLM: 1. Health
education. WA590 R966h]
RA440.R87   613'.07'1073   75-12809
ISBN 0-8106-1354-9

PREFACE

The Joint Committee on Health Problems in Education of the National Education Association and the American Medical Association is pleased to present this sixth edition of a pioneering venture in health education that was first initiated in 1924.

This edition represents a distinct departure from the previous five publications. A single author rather than an editor and many contributors was contracted to write the manuscript. As in previous editions, the Joint Committee through a sub-committee suggested the format and was actively involved in its development and completion. This book represents the creativity and humaneness of the writer as he sought to capture and interpret the concerns of the Committee. It has been a highly coordinated effort and venture that hopefully will be recognized and accepted as professional progress for Joint Committee publications.

The sixth edition emphasizes the behavioral and valuing aspects of health in education and the community. It is a philosophical-based rather than a how-to-do-it type of publication. It presents current health problems and issues through its illustrations; it considers the various curriculum aspects of health instruction without exploring all the nitty-gritty details. It is a resource book for teachers, prospective teachers, physicians, school nurses, public health education personnel and others in the allied and school health fields; it focuses on future decisions rather than discussing the traditional and status quo situations.

Health Education is a companion volume to *School Health Services* and *Healthful School Environment,* first published in 1953 and 1957 respectively. These volumes offer a comprehensive view of the total school health program—education, service and environment—and will assist in answering many of today's health problems in education. This sixth edition of *Health Education* is offered in the confident belief that it suggests a refreshing, humanistic direction for education—the third part of the triad of the total health program in both schools and communities.

The Joint Committee and its parent organizations, the National Education Association and the American Medical Association, wish to express sincere appreciation to Dr. Robert Russell for his wisdom and perception as reflected in these pages as well as his tremendous skill and personal involvement that give this publication its unique flavor and quality.

Charles H. McMullen, M.D.
Chairman 1972-1973
Nancy Willis
Chairman 1973-1974
Marcia F. Curry, M.D.
Chairman 1974-1975

Quoted passages in this book may use the pronoun "he" to denote an abstract individual, e.g., "the student." We have not attempted to alter this usage, although we currently use "she/he" in such instances.

NEA Publishing

TABLE OF CONTENTS

Chapter I   Health Education . . . A Book 9

Chapter II   Health . . . and Education 13

Chapter III   Health in the U.S.A.—Mid-1970's 33

Chapter IV   The Nature of the Learners 49

Chapter V   Health Education: Science and Non-Science 75

Chapter VI   Attitudes and Other Affectors of Behavior 87

Chapter VII   Risk-Taking 103

Chapter VIII   Getting High 117

Chapter IX   Health and Health Education in Ecological
                   Perspective 127

Chapter X   Some March to Different Drums 143

Chapter XI   Curriculum Development 151

Chapter XII   Teaching-Learning Strategies 171

Chapter XIII   Materials and Resources 189

Chapter XIV   So What Have We Accomplished?
                   (Sometimes Tabbed Evaluation) 215

Chapter XV   Health Education Beyond the School 231

Chapter XVI   Some Future for Health Education 241

Joint Committee on Health Problems in Education of the
    National Education Association and the American Medical
                   Association 251

Chapter I

Health Education...
A Book

HEALTH EDUCATION. Health Education? Health Education! The term represents both a discipline or field of study and a profession or field of work. The profession is one that centers on improving communications about health matters and motivating people to life-styles that result in better total functioning.

Because health education is a discipline, books are written about it. This is one of those books. It is offered as a resource book for educators, a text for health teacher education and for preparation of community health educators, health service personnel such as nurses and physicians, school personnel and others with concern for children of school age. It is not written for youngsters, high school and younger. Remember this when you are tempted to ask, "Couldn't he have used fewer examples from sensitive and controversial areas?"

A FURTHER EXPLANATION: This is not what most readers would call a traditional textbook. The Joint Committee on Health Problems in Education . . . perused and evaluated at least ten current books describing this discipline and profession and found many of these adequate to excellent. Most were written in good, solid textbook style. So the Committee's charge was that this not be a cookbook, not another how-to book, because another one would appear to be redundant. Instead, it is a philosophical treatise . . . dealing more with what and why than with when, where, and how. It is a text with a future orientation . . . not so much in the form of predictions about what's coming as it is an extension of ideas, programs, and present phenomena into the future, including exploration of alternative actions and reactions. The valuing process emerges again and again throughout the pages . . . for how and what we value strongly influence what we are and do . . . and what we shall be and do.

As American culture shifts and changes, health education must respond through discovering and developing and using approaches that achieve maximum communication . . . and learning. Many Americans have some values and attitudes in common, but there are many more differences among U.S. folk than health education has assumed in the past. Effectiveness may increase with the realization and serious consideration of individual and group differences.

IS SUCH A BOOK NEEDED? Some of you who are well-established in the field and accustomed to traditional texts may honestly ask, "Is this book really necessary?" The honest basis for a positive defense is that perhaps the field needs to explore some new ways of thinking about health education, its needs and opportunities. At present there is no book that examines the field in light of this philosophy. The call is for some unexpected words, some unusual phrases, some unlikely sentences, and some provocative cases and examples. Hopefully, these will help open minds and serve up ideas for open minds.

NON-TRADITIONAL RESOURCE BOOK. Typically a resource book has an index. This resource book has none. In general, each chapter develops ideas in a context, making rather inappropriate the looking up of such specific terms as concept, contraceptive, or controlling variables.

HEALTH EDUCATION-HUMAN STORIES. The examples appearing in the following chapter present the notion that health education in schools is a part of health education that begins in early childhood and continues throughout life. The school health educator often has certain unique health education opportunities, but there is less and less reason to see this form of health education as being greatly different from other forms. The examples are meant to emphasize that the health education story is essentially a human story. Health makes a poor abstract concept, because it really is about Jim and Carolyn and Arturo and old Mrs. Jefferson and how they function. Health education is also about Mr. Adams and his class of sixth graders, what Rosemary tells Marcia, and about the debate teams headed by Joseph and Alice. In these pages, the norm is that principles shall not just be stated; instead, principles shall derive from understandable human behavior with which you may be able to identify. Then the principles lead on to further illustrations of how real people might function or even cope adequately or better.

SPIRITUAL DIMENSIONS. In addition to the expected dimensions of well-being that encompass health—physical, mental, emotional, social—the approach in this book includes the spiritual. This book makes no case for any particular spiritual dimension, but merely acknowledges that many human beings, educators and educatees, believe in such a dimension. There is no assertion that "spiritual" and "religious" are synonymous.

ACCURACY AND COMMUNICATION. Undoubtedly some people whose education is in one of the health disciplines will study or browse through these pages. Likewise, some readers will be educators with less medical-scientific background. Health practitioners learn specialized vocabularies to insure accuracy in communication with one another; so do educators. Yet such vocabularies also create an in-group; those within communicate, while those not in do not understand. Health education . . . and this book . . . must, at certain times, give up semantic accuracy to enhance broader communication. At other times, it tries to enlarge learners' vocabularies and working concepts.

If you at least glanced at the table of contents, you spotted some chapters that seem quite traditional and expected. There is "The Nature of the Learners," "Curriculum Development," and a familiar one, "Materials and Resources." Although one is entitled "So What Have We Accomplished?" it is on the old familiar topic of evaluation. So there is a core of traditional strength and continuity. But there are some reasonably unusual headings also, like "Risk-Taking," "Getting High," ". . . Ecological Perspective," and "Some March to Different Drums."

STYLE. Even where content is orthodox, the style may depart from the textbook model. For example, you should pick up rather quickly a departure from the usual practice of always using "he" as the pronoun for either male or female. It can be argued that this simplifies the reading, but we're increasingly conscious of what else it can connote. She/he, him/her have been interspersed not to confuse the reader but to point out that those who learn include both females and males.

THE WRITER IS AN I. From time to time you will encounter such unexpected phrases as "I had an experience. . . . ," "as I analyze this. . . . ," ". . . it seems to me. . . ."—all anathema to a professional textbook. Previous editions of this book were the product of committees. Although this edition was planned by and received consultation from the Joint Committee, it is essentially a single-author effort. But even so, the expected style would be to keep it entirely impersonal. Most of what is written here is not just my opinion; but, in honesty, when something is, I am inclined to identify it as such. If "I am I" and "you are you" in the book, it has the potential for being more like a conversation than a formal lecture.

Health education is an exciting field, full of potential for both personal satisfaction and service to others. The latter part of that statement is reasonably verifiable; the rest is rather subjective. But I feel it, and I hope I can communicate it . . . along with the objective facts and ideas. This book may irritate you . . . or, happily, the feeling may be more like stimulate or excite. Whatever it is, hopefully you will remember some of it . . . even quote it. . . .

A FOREWORD? Perceptive, veteran text readers probably are saying, "This is like a preface or a foreword. How come it was put as Chapter One?" Because the Joint Committee, many of whom admit they do not regularly read forewords, felt it was an essential orientation to the fifteen chapters that follow.

Chapter II

Health...
and Education

WHAT IS HEALTH, ANYWAY? Health is . . . feelin' good when you get up in the morning . . . it's feelin' good even when you miss two spelling words . . . it's enjoying the freedom of recess but not really minding going back to try to learn something more . . . it's climbing a tree to look at a bird's nest . . . it's feeding your cat, even when nobody reminds you . . . it's being able to play hard, with both kids you like and don't . . . it's feelin' good about goin' to bed, 'cause there'll be more good and fun things to do tomorrow.

It's being satisfied with the body you have and yet wanting to maintain and even improve its condition and appearance . . . it's being satisfied with where your head's at and yet willing to experience and learn new things and even change your ideas . . . it's being satisfied with what sex you are and yet being real interested in what the opposite is like . . . it's knowing you are an individual but getting real satisfaction out of relating to others and not necessarily being No. 1.

It's getting satisfaction from your work without having your whole identity being what you do . . . it's getting married because you want to and are ready to and then keeping a balance between the real joys of marriage and the real pains of living closely with a person who isn't like you, in certain ways . . . it's taking care of a body that's been functioning quite a few years, balancing off what you can do with what you no longer can.

And when you get older, it's living with a certain amount of pain and discomfort without being a self-centered martyr and yet without letting it interfere too much with the enjoyable things you still can do . . . it's living with the fact that what you'll hear from many of your friends is about their infirmities . . . it's making new friends when it would be easier just to remain lonely . . . it's accepting the fact that you have to be dependent on others in some ways but still doing as much as you can for yourself . . . it's realizing that your dependence is a means by which younger persons can get the satisfaction of being helpful to someone in need.

Come on, now, why begin with these when there are probably more than a dozen good, solid, respectable definitions of health? Because a definition means most to the person or persons who devised it, something a bit less to people who have had fairly comparable experiences, and very little to folks without the experiences condensed into and interpreted by the definition. A definition is a deduction from data, a descriptive principle derived from experiences, actual and vicarious, practical and academic. The World Health Organization (or, more accurately, those persons who represented it in 1947) defines health as

> A state of complete physical, mental, and social well-being, and not merely the absence of disease or infirmity.

Vast numbers of health professionals have (willingly or unwillingly) attempted to memorize these nineteen words over the last twenty-five years, but one wonders whether it continues to be the way they define health as they live and work beyond the academic classroom. Would this definition have helped the four people who described health in more living terms at the beginning of this discussion?

As a matter of fact, without some prompting from this concept, the description would more likely have dwelt on physical conditions . . . perhaps even on absences, such as "I have no cavities," "My nose isn't stuffy anymore," "I lost the ten pounds I gained over the holidays," "My feet don't itch" . . . and so on. The most common reference for which the word health is a cue is the physical body; in the last few decades the mental dimension has become a more obvious portion of health for more people. The social, however, is a dimension of well-being that most folks would have to be coaxed to include as health.

HOW MANY DIMENSIONS TO THE WHOLE PERSON? The World Health Organization definition deserves the credit for giving some tangibility to the holistic concept of health—physical, mental and social well-being. While three is a handy number, the criticism can be leveled that this concept is too simplistic. Mental, for example, must include both the intellectual (what one knows) and the emotional (how one feels). Most health professionals would agree that this is a lumping of potentially dissonant aspects of the human being in health education. For years, we have separated knowledge and attitudes and said things like, "She knows that she shouldn't smoke, but she doesn't feel like quitting" or "He knows the potential value of the buckled-up seatbelt, but his attitude is 'It won't happen to me.' " Thus, mental well-being may be too broad a concept.

Since publicly supported education is not supposed to support any established religion or interfere with the free exercise thereof, and since health has been associated with the establishment of medicine (where the recommended way of viewing life is naturalistic-scientific), it has been the general policy of orthodox health education not to acknowledge a spiritual dimension to well-being. If the spiritual portion of well-being has to do the acknowledging and relating to a power greater than self (supernatural or not so), recognizing an aspect of self called spirit or soul, and doing things that benefit others more than self, probably many more Americans would consider this an important dimension of health than would not. Some would argue that this is just a part of mental health or social well-being. Others would counter that it is only true if social is also really mental . . . or if mental is a part of physical. Others would say that it is an affirmation of good mental health or good social relationships. Still others would have to call this the spiritual—related to, but definitely different from all other definitions. The point here is not to decide—for everyone—whether there is or is not a spiritual dimension of well-being. Rather, it is to admit that while many people deny its existence and necessity, many others affirm it and some would certainly rank it as the prime criterion of good health.

Oberteuffer [1] has suggested aesthetic well-being as another dimension possibly different enough from the ones already described to be acknowledged. This would involve the relative capacity to appreciate beauty in its many forms, as perceived through any sense or any combination of senses.

A STATE OR A FUNCTION? The major point is that whether well-being has three dimensions—or four, five, or six, or more—*health is a condition of the totality of human beings.*

The exact nature of this condition has been questioned by some thoughtful health professionals, including Pollock who criticized the concept of health as "a *state* of . . . well-being," arguing that it "suffers from a certain circularity in that it defines health as a state of well-being which is to say that health is a state of health." [2] But more importantly, she argues that health should be seen not so much as a state but as the quality of functioning of the organism, in all its complexity. As an academic argument this is a good one, but let's use the statements at the beginning of the chapter as a means of deciding. *It's feelin' good even when you miss two spelling words. . . . It's being satisfied with the body you have. . . . It's getting satisfaction from your work. . . .* these all refer to some specific or general function, but they also seem to be describing a state of being that applies at the time of speaking. *It's climbing a tree. . . . It's keeping a balance between the joys and pains . . . of marriage. . . . It's living with a certain amount of pain. . . .* these seem clearly to involve more process or functioning. Perhaps, then, health is both a state of well-being assessable at any moment in time and a quality of functioning over some period of time. Health can be described both as a state and as a functioning.

---

[1] Oberteuffer, Delbert and Beyrer, Mary K., *School Health Education* (Fourth Edition). New York: Harper & Row, Publishers, 1966. pg. 39.

[2] Oberteuffer, Delbert, Harrelson, Orvis A., and Pollock, Marion B., *School Health Education* (Fifth Edition). New York: Harper & Row, Publishers, 1972. pg. 10.

ABSOLUTE OR RELATIVE? Another interesting critical point that Pollock raises is that of defining health in terms that are, practically speaking, unattainable—i.e., complete physical, mental and social well-being. What is the point of characterizing health as a state that no one is likely to achieve? Shouldn't it be thought of as a relative condition, requiring a modifier of some sort—very poor, lousy, so-so, good, excellent . . . even perfect? The issue is not, of course, whether people (or societies) display degrees of this characteristic—this should be obviously so; rather it is whether these degrees are spelled-out or simply understood. It is unlikely that the folks who devised the W.H.O. definition or anyone who approves of and uses it would assert that everyone who does not have this triad of complete well-being is unhealthy. It is more likely that they would simply name the ideal and assume that approximations of it can be called healthy. For example, a woman may say she has a happy marriage, even though the relationship has its moments of distress. She just says it is happy even though it is possible that it is not complete happiness.

The point of all this is that while the criticism by Pollock and colleagues Oberteuffer and Harrelson evokes a preference for defining health as "the condition of the organism that measures the degree to which its aggregate powers are able to function" [3] the meaning, as translated by living, functioning beings, would be basically the same. One interpretation needs the relative quality stated; the other assumes it without statement.

HEALTH—WEATHER AND CLIMATE. Another way of viewing health as a state and a function might be compared to the use of the term weather. If I should interpret the often-posed query, "How are you?" as "How is your health?", how should I generalize from a longer time period? At this moment I have a cold, with a stuffy head, running nose and incipient cough, a condition of less than supreme well-being. But the quality of my well-being over the years of these middle 40's is excellent. Which is the state of my health? Which is the quality of my functioning? Probably both. We use the word "weather" to describe the state and process of temperature, precipitation, air movement, etc., for yesterday, today and tomorrow; we substitute the word "climate" for a generalization about the weather of a particular region over a longer time span. Realistically, for our present concern, we have no separate distinction; health stands for both.

SOME WAYS OF BALANCING. Can you stand one more complexity? We might agree that complete physical, mental and social well-being translated into functioning would be doing everything just right. This would mean things like eating a balanced diet daily, not smoking, exer-

---

[3] Ibid.

cising daily, consciously making new friends, controlling anger at a time when its expression would hurt others . . . a theoretically perfect balance of uncountable do's and don'ts. Such a paragon, existing in theory, would have to be called healthy. But what about us real people? Some of us earn the appellation healthy by balancing somewhat extreme behaviors, while others approach it through more moderate behavior. Molly is a housewife, mother, writer, and civic worker who does some of each nearly every day, successfully dividing her time, talents and duties; Joan has the same combination of roles, but she may write for two full days, clean the house once a week, work diligently on a civic project for a full week, etc., and if her family accepts this and appreciates her life-style it can be an equally healthy approach. Molly and Tom make it a point to go out for dinner and an evening of entertainment at least once every two weeks; Keith and Joan rarely go out for an evening like this, preferring to save their resources for a week or a two-week stay at a resort they both will enjoy.

Some folks seek balance through mixing desirables. Then, some folks mix desirables and undesirables in different ways. For example, three professional men all appear to function equally well in their jobs: Charlie controls his weight well, but smokes and exercises sporadically, while Ray is obese and smokes, but exercises heavily and regularly, and Dick controls his weight and doesn't smoke, but exercises as little as possible. Another for instance: Charlene and Dorothy leave a party about the same time; Charlene drives home after drinking all evening with her seat belt securely fastened, while Dorothy has had no alcohol but drives home sitting on her seat belt.

Let's face it: everyone tends to prefer to define real health more in terms of the way she/he functions than in ways that would seem to make her/him seem deviant. Naturally moderate people usually would favor equating health with moderation in all things. Less moderate people, whose lives involve taking more risks, usually see health as the effective mixing of these risks. Very immoderate people might see health more in terms of the intensity of experiencing life, even if some of these experiences would be judged detrimental by the more moderate.

Is this a fair analogy for health in general? Can we accept a range of ways in which people deal with the challenge of functioning as a living person and consider all of them healthy? Or, as someone's behavior displeases us or affects us in some uncomfortable way, do we tend to constrict our judgment as to what is healthy? Perhaps it's time for an example with the use of mood modifiers. With the foregoing conclusion as a premise, the analogy would be that a man who never uses alcoholic beverage or any drug sustances in any form (except for medical purposes) would tend to feel that his position would be healthiest for all. However, the healthier position would be the one in which he realizes the strength of his own life-style but acknowledges that some people might have different values and thus could function well even though they were not abstainers. The extreme broad-minded position would be accepting the fact that some young people's view of life values risk-taking and experimenting in such ways as to make taking of hallucinogenic drugs appear to be healthy behavior. However, such an open-minded abstaining gentleman might well demur from this general live-and-let-live position if his wife should be the one to start drinking, or when his daughter is the one to try tripping with lysergic acid diethylamide, or when he is mugged by a young man trying to maintain his equilibrium with heroin.

A GENERALIZATION. Is there a generalization concerning health behavior that is important to educating about health? Very probably. It would be something like this: the most free position one could take would be accepting any behavior as potentially healthy for the individual, irrespective of how it might have affected others previously. The most restrained position would be one of defining healthy behavior as being like one's own and as one feels one should behave. Defections from broad-mindedness are the result of experiences that make one believe some behaviors are going to be harmful to oneself or to others whom one cares about. An open-minded position may thus pose the dilemma that you care for many people and their well-being, which can be maintained only by taking away their freedom of choice, which you also value highly. Well, we could ruminate upon these complexities and variations on a theme interminably, but sooner or later we must try to see how health is related to health education.

HEALTH AND HEALTH EDUCATION

HEALTH EDUCATION. Everyone's education in health begins at a very tender age and continues until the last capacity and desire to think and remember ebb away.

- Health education means gaining new knowledge, having knowledge already acquired reinforced, and having ideas learned previously presented in a new or different way so that they are now more understandable and usable.
- Health education means developing new attitudes, having present attitudes reinforced, and having other present attitudes modified.
- Health education means trying new behaviors, continuing to act as before with new conviction, and modifying some behaviors.

When I first learned these three components of health education, I learned them as a list of three things, like "See no evil, hear no evil, speak no evil" or "Winken, Blinken, and Nod." I learned that these are measured by knowledge tests, attitude scales, and health awareness tests (later caller health practice tests—then behavior inventories). More recently, I worked on a curriculum project where we were concerned with the cognitive domain, the affective domain, and the action domain. Though each is a separate component, it has become increasingly evident to me that in the totality of health education any individual experiences, they clearly interact and should be represented thus:

ATTITUDES   KNOWLEDGE

BEHAVIOR

with the strong implication that each affects the other and that the interrelationships are moving and dynamic.

As an example, let's follow Ted and some of his encounters with health education involving cigarette smoking.

Age 3—asks for puff on Dad's cigarette . . . is told smoking is not for children . . . has two attitudes—smoking looks like fun and it isn't for me to do

Age 8—sneaks one of Dad's cigarettes and smokes it . . . likes the feeling of blowing the smoke but not of inhaling . . . knows that he must sneak smokes if he is to continue . . . doesn't like to do sneaky things

Age 14—learns in health class and from his athletic coach that smoking hinders athletic performance . . . feels like smoking is a "cool" thing to do, but feels he should follow training rules while on an athletic team . . . does not smoke at all during athletic season . . . has an occasional cigarette with friends out-of-season

Age 18—knows long-range possible effects of smoking on the body . . . is no longer on athletic team and feels like doing what he was prevented from doing—smoking . . . begins to smoke regularly, about a pack a day

Age 24—moves to a large city . . . knows that breathing city air is equivalent to smoking what he now averages . . . does not feel like doubling his risk . . . stops smoking

Age 26—is transferred to a smaller city . . . has gained twenty pounds in two years . . . has learned that overweight and smoking are comparable contributing factors to illness . . . has missed smoking . . . decides to start again

Age 40—physical exam shows high blood pressure . . . knows smoking is now making him more vulnerable to ill-health . . . has several friends who say they can't quit . . . feels like he does not want to be controlled by a smoking habit like they are . . . quits smoking for good

In some instances Ted's attitude determined behavior; in others his knowledge affected how he felt and what he did; in others he learned from doing; in others, attitudes were affected by behavior . . . and so on.

CONTENT AND PROCESS. In addition to illustrating the many interactions among knowledge, attitudes, and behavior, the above vignettes
concerning Ted and his smoking also serve as examples of one of the
most important understandings about health education: it is both content
and process. It is what you learn and how you learn it. It is learning,
remembering and being able to utilize ideas, concepts, facts, feelings
and actions . . . and, at the same time, it is learning how to learn. Some
humans learn rather efficiently . . . others can learn only in relatively few
ways. Much of what is learned is forgotten . . . or at least seems so to
to the conscious mind. An important perspective, then, is that encouraging a person to learn something new may be also encouraging
her/him to forget something already learned, related or unrelated to that
being learned. So, how does health education take place?

- Mrs. Dawes tells her 15-month-old repeatedly not to go out in the
  street because of the danger of cars, and she spanks him when he
  does.

- Six-year-old Martin tells his little sister to brush her teeth with the
  fluoride toothpaste (he uses a brand name) so she may not have
  any cavities . . . like the one he just had filled.

- Claudia and many of her soon-to-be classmates take a pre-school
  physical exam at the school and learn that some shots are necessary
  to keep you from getting sick; by taking the shots they also learn
  that they really hurt very little.

- Pablo and his classmates learn that while school will help them
  learn to speak English, their Spanish language is an important one,
  and they may speak it at times and even help their teacher improve
  her use of it—an important tangential lesson in mental health.

- Julie and five seventh-grade classmates are a committee to survey
  and analyze all the billboard and advertising in their part of town
  that relates to health; they are learning to observe, to compare
  judgments, and to be more aware of all that is health-related.

- Timmy's ninth-grade class is having a mock trial on a character
  called Practice O'Smoking, and Timmy is the defense attorney who
  must argue convincingly that smoking should be free to be utilized
  by people if they so choose.

- Angie, 15, goes to a party with an older boy; during the party he
  takes some speed, and she learns, the hard trial-and-error way, how
  to cope with a boy who is hopped up and physically and sexually
  aggressive.

- Mike sprains his ankle badly playing football, and during the recovery process he learns a great deal from the trainer about how
  ankles function and how one can encourage them to heal rapidly.

- Jill has learned in health and driver education class and through community health education media that it is dangerous to drive after drinking . . . and she never has; after a recent party, however, her date had a lot to drink, but still drove her and then himself home without any accident, so now she has another piece of information. . . .
- Frank is a combat soldier whose buddy is hit by grenade fragments; Frank remembers all the appropriate first aid treatment and he administers it quickly and well, but still has the experience of seeing his buddy die, despite all he could do.
- Millie is afraid she's going to become pregnant. She knows a lot about how it happens and how it can be prevented, but she's afraid she doesn't know enough. Her college health professor reinforces much of what she knows, corrects a few things, adds some new information, and the small group discussions give her a chance to have several important questions answered without embarrassment, and she is no longer afraid . . . from ignorance.
- Helen is a young adult and overweight. She follows her doctor's diet and takes the prescribed pills, without good results, so she reads all she can on dieting, talks to friends, and is now on a diet that was successful with a friend she trusts . . . and is losing weight.
- Duke is middle-aged and has recently had a serious heart attack. During his recovery period he learns much from his physician and recommended reading about what brought this on and how he should live now and for the rest of his life; he is not at all hesitant about talking to younger men whose life-styles and body care seem to be about like his before the attack, urging them to consider modifying "before it happens to them."
- Grandma Rudd is 85 years old, healthy, and spry. Her physician is a young man, and she consults him and has him check her regularly, but continues to use and tell others about her own potions and medications that have helped her live actively this long. She respects medicine, but she feels that many of the old-time treatments are good, too, and less expensive . . . and might be forgotten if she doesn't pass them along to others.

If these are selected examples of health education, what do they tell us about the content and process of this important human activity? Let's recall that health involves the totality of the functioning person—social, mental (intellectual and emotional) and physical . . . perhaps even spiritual and aesthetic. Let's also recall that health education involves knowledge, attitudes and behavior. And also . . .

- *Health education goes on at all ages.* Very small children are told and conditioned about things parents believe they should and should not do, but it isn't long before one child knows something that another should know . . . so he tells him. This goes on all the way through life, then, to Duke and Grandma Rudd . . . both still learning and still teaching.

- *Health education usually begins in the home,* and is usually based on "authority knows best." However, the desire of the individual to learn what one wants to know soon asserts itself, and learning by authoritative fiat must be supplemented, perhaps nearly replaced, by deciding for oneself. Health education, nevertheless, has a strong authority base to it, which sometimes helps and sometimes hinders its effectiveness.

- *Health education takes place in peer groups,* and between siblings and good friends. Here authority is supplemented by trust and friendship, with a more personal element involved in helping someone learn something he/she did not know. Academic health educators frequently condemn or ridicule such exchanges because they may be inaccurate.

- *Health education comes from experiencing environments.* The physicial exam provides a setting for some important learning; the training room where the sprained ankle is being treated is another; the doctor's office or the hospital room for the coronary recoverer are others. The health education classroom in the school can be such an experiencing environment.

- *Health education comes from experiences.* Having an injection is a way of knowing what a shot is like and probably affects how one feels about it. Having to cope with a date who is aggressively high on amphetamines is a way of knowing what drug abuse is and undoubtedly will affect one's feeling about it. It also might reveal what one's own values really are. Getting home unscathed with a drinking driver may help teach a dubiously healthful but sometimes true lesson: a person does an unhealthful thing and no ill-effect comes of it. The experiences of a child who does not know English well in being allowed to use her/his own language at times may be a positive experience in building sense of self and more probably prevents that development of inferiority and resentment feelings which certainly skews an individual's functioning toward the unhappy and unproductive.

- *Health education involves the reciprocal teaching-learning process,* because teaching someone something she/he doesn't know may be an encouragement to learn something further from someone else.

- *Health education often involves working with others,* observing, analyzing, and comparing observations and judgments.

- *Health education should be a means of contact* between the school and the community in which it is located. The student lives in both school and community, and should have as many experiences as possible which suggest that these are not completely separate worlds.

- *Health education involves simulating life situations,* such as having a learner defend in a trial the dubious practice of smoking, requiring some faith that the experience of honest inquiry rather than apparently safer propagandizing leads to better personal decisions.

- *Health education involves capitalizing on the teachable moment.* When an athlete has a sprained ankle or an active, busy man has a heart attack, motivations for learning why and "What do I do now?" are often very high. Professional health personnel like physicians, nurses, trainers, etc., have many such opportunities, but so do parents and friends, with each other.

- *Health education should deal with the seeming contradictions* between academic learning, such as "drunken drivers have significantly more fatal accidents than non-drinking drivers," and life experiences, like "he was drunk but he drove me home without an accident." Some people who brush their teeth faithfully and skillfully still develop caries; some people who eat ravenously do not get fat; some people select a marriage partner with great care and are still unhappy.

- *Health education may involve the experience of failing,* as with Frank who did skillfully everything he knew to do and still his buddy died. Our apparent failure . . . the girl won't take a drink and the boy she really likes won't invite her out again . . . the girl who walks home rather than ride with a drunk and gets harangued for being late . . . In other words, one may know and remember the best thing to do, but it sometimes does not appear to work.

- *Health education often involves encouraging fear* as a motivator to learning and then abating the fear with some positive alternatives. Education of small children about safety in relation to traffic usually has some fear component—cars can hurt you. This should then motivate the fledgling learner to learn what to do to prevent such potential harm. Martin also is trying to scare his sister into brushing to avoid cavities. Fear to motivate; then positive action to allay the cause of fear.

- *Health education involves maintaining a balance* between the pronouncements of physicians and the scientific community and the experiences of people as they live and perceive life. Science has made tremendous contributions to the betterment of human life, but science is best in studying simple, controllable things and situations, and is most frustrated with any study of humankind in totality in community with other total beings.

MUTUAL LEARNING. This all might be summed up by crying that health education is potentially best when it involves mutual learning. The learners learn from the teacher, but the teacher also learns something from them; learners learn from each other; learners learn from the community and its experiences, and the community learns from the learners. A hopefully never-ending process.

SCHOOL HEALTH EDUCATION. What responsibility do the schools have for health education? With some regularity over the past four score or so years, statements have become part of the public domain that affirm that in American society the school does have as a goal the encouragement of health in learners.

One of the earliest affirmations was the formation in 1885 of a professional organization, The American Association for the Advancement of Physical Education, which was to join with the Health Division of the National Education Association and become the American Association for Health, Physical Education and Recreation. (It has since become the American Alliance for Health, Physical Education and Recreation.) As a department of the N.E.A. it was responsible for much early encouragement of school health programs. In 1911 the Joint Committee on Health Problems in Education of the National Education Association and the American Medical Association emerged, presaging regularly published resolutions and materials melding the judgments of both medical and educational professionals.

The Commission on the Reorganization of Secondary Education (N.E.A.) in its 1918 report [4] announced the Seven Cardinal Principles or outcomes of education: health, command of fundamental processes, worthy home-membership, vocation, civic education, worthy use of leisure time, and ethical character. So, if health is to be a cardinal outcome of their efforts with youngsters, the schools presumably should give some instructional time to this aspect of human life. Twenty years later, The Educational Policies Commission developed a statement, *The Purposes of Education in American Democracy,*[5] which came to be seen as a classic, describing desired pupil outcomes in each of four groups of educational objectives: self-realization, human relationship, economic efficiency, and civic responsibility. In discussing education for self-

---

[4] Commission on the Reorganization of Secondary Education, *Cardinal Principles of Secondary Education.* Washington, D.C.: Department of the Interior, Bureau of Education, Bulletin 1918, no. 35, 1918. pp. 11-15.

[5] Educational Policies Commission, National Education Association of the United States and the American Association of School Administrators, *The Purposes of Education in American Democracy.* Washington, D.C.: National Education Association, 1938. pg. 47.

realization, the Commission says that the health-educated person is characterized as follows:

1. *The educated person understands the basic facts concerning health and disease.* Health is a factor that conditions our success in all our undertakings, personal and social. For that reason schools properly place great emphasis on health as an outcome of education.

2. *The educated person protects his own health and that of his dependents.* Knowing what is necessary for maintaining health in body and mind, the educated person so conducts his life as to respect these great rules of the game. He tries to secure competent medical advice and treatment for himself and his family, with special attention to the early discovery and treatment of remediable defects and a systematic plan of health inventory and illness prevention.

3. *The educated person works to improve the health of the community.* The interests of the educated person in the field of health are comprehensive. That which he desires for himself in this field, the educated person desires also for others, knowing that health is one commodity that is increased in proportion as it is shared. Especially in a democracy, the educated person will cherish a sincere interest in maintaining the health standards of the entire community.[6]

A few years later, a Special Committee of the American Council on Education reported on *What the High Schools Ought to Teach* and stated that ". . . there must be a place in any program of general education for a course in personal problems. Perhaps the most urgent of these is that of maintaining one's physical and mental health."[7]

Seven years went by and a White House Conference on Education, attended by representatives of many segments of society, sent a report to the President that answered the question, "What should our schools accomplish?" Of the 14 competencies that schools should help each student develop, the following (starting with number 3) have some degree of relationship to health and health education as both content and process.[8]

3. Understanding the civic rights and responsibilities and knowledge of American institutions

---

[6] Ibid., pp. 60-63.

[7] Special Committee on the Secondary School Curriculum, *What the High Schools Ought to Teach.* Washington, D.C.: American Council on Education, 1940. pp. 24-25.

[8] The Committee for the White House Conference on Education. *A Report to the President.* Washington, D.C.: Superintendent of Documents, Government Printing Office, 1956.

4. Respect and appreciation for human values and for the beliefs of others

5. Ability to think and evaluate constructively and creatively

6. Effective work habits and self-discipline

7. Social competence as a contributing member of his family and community

8. Ethical behavior based on a sense of moral and spiritual values

9. Intellectual curiosity and eagerness for life-long learning

10. Physical and mental health

11. Wise use of time, including constructive leisure pursuits

12. Understanding of the physical world and man's relation to it as represented through basic knowledge of the sciences

13. An awareness of our relationships with the world community

As the 1960's began, the Educational Policies Commission published a document called *The Central Purpose of American Education,* defining that as the development of the thinking person. Regarding health they wrote:

> Each of the school's . . . objectives can be better achieved as pupils develop (the ability to think) and learn to apply it to all the problems that face them. *Health,* for example, depends on a reasoned awareness of the value of mental and physical fitness and of the means by which it can be developed and maintained. Fitness . . . requires that the individual understand the connection between health, nutrition, activity, and environment, and that he take action to improve his mental and physical condition.[9]

During the 1960's, the U.S. experienced a sense of inferiority regarding some aspects of its educational capability, in some sense a kind of last gasp of the cold war mentality or "Egad, we're not as good as they are . . . and we must be better." This flurry of educational upgrading centered mostly in mathematics, sciences, and foreign languages. Though professions of concern for health education still broke forth from time to time, there never was any tangible support by the Federal Government to match that for the aforementioned areas of learning.

One interesting happening merits mention here, however. The School Health Education Study (to be described in Chapter XI) came into being because a couple of prominent and action-oriented public health physicians convinced a private foundation to support a nationwide status study of health education. A published synthesis of the research in the field and the organization and planning of a concept-

---

[9] Educational Policies Commission of the National Education Association and the American Association of School Administrators, *The Central Purpose of American Education.* Washington, D.C.: National Education Association, 1961. pg. 5

based curriculum resulted. One of these physicians, Granville Larimore was, prior to this successful funding operation, a member and chairman of the Joint Committee on Health Problems in Education of the National Education Association and the American Medical Association and was deeply influenced by that experience. The Study, after it was established through support from the Bronfman Foundation, became even more unique when its completion and dissemination were assured through a grant from a private industrial firm, the 3M Company of St. Paul, Minnesota. So while health education received no significant federal attention during the 1960's, a number of states and school districts made attempts to implement some updated programs.

THE COALITION . . . AND THEN THE PRESIDENT'S COMMITTEE. The 1970's auditioned and became operational, and the profession experienced a pair of related firsts: the President of the United States, Richard M. Nixon, appointed in September, 1971 a Committee on Health Education. Before this Committee even organized, however, eight professional groups, seeing the potential future need for less splintered and factious health education activities, joined in "A Working Agreement for a Coalition of National Health Education Organizations" in December 1971.[10] The Coalition consisted of the following with identifiable health educator memberships:

- American Alliance for Health, Physical Education and Recreation
- American College Health Association
- American Public Health Association
- Conference of State and Territorial Directors of Public Health Education
- Society of State Directors of Health, Physical Education and Recreation
- Society for Public Health Education, Inc.
- American School Health Association

Its "Working Agreement" promised that on a long-range basis it would sponsor a periodic review and reporting of research in health education and would encourage cooperative communication among groups with common purposes. As a shorter task it would make an assessment of the President's Committee's final report and then would provide leadership for a national audit of the report and for the follow-up that surely would be necessary.

Meanwhile, the seventeen-member President's Committee on Health Education, including representatives from health education and several

---

[10] "The Coalition in Chicago," *SOPHE News & Views*, 3:3–4 (no. 3), May 1974.

portions of the health care industry, from business, industry, and labor, came together and set its course of action. The committee was charged with describing the state of the art of health education of the public in the U.S. today, defining needs, establishing goals and priorities proposing recommendations and developing a plan for the implementation of its recommendations. A more complete description of the work of the Committee, its recommendations to the President and the possible effects appears in a later chapter.

NO REAL MANDATE. All of this (and particularly the earlier, historical affirmations) would seem to suggest that the schools have a fairly clear mandate to be active in health education. Not really so. American public schools have typically been a vacillating mixture of institutions—classic educational and pragmatic social (custodial, too, unfortunately). As classic educational institutions, they are to follow the lead of European schools and American private schools, that is, teaching the basic skills of reading, writing, and arithmetic in order that students might study subjects such as English grammar, composition and literature, foreign languages, mathematics, physical and life sciences, history, and geography. The assumption behind these curriculum priorities is that the home, the church, and the community are the real influencing factors in a youngster's life, and they are responsible for teaching about living life . . . about aspects of personal behavior and about vocational skills. The school is basically to teach those things most youngsters would not learn well from their parents, church, and community.

However, as schools became universal and compulsory, it became obvious that here was a captive audience of malleable youth, and since communities and society supported the schools, they should be utilized for the benefit of society. Further, as American society came to include more and more diverse elements (ethnic groups), segments of the society became more alarmed about the diverse things youngsters were learning at home (or that they were not learning at all) and so pressures on the school to include teaching about issues crucial to the stability of society began to mount. Jefferson asserted that "if a nation expects to be ignorant and free, in a state of civilization, it expects what never was and never will be." [11] Jefferson, however, assumed that the voting franchise would go only to those with education and therefore the maintenance of freedom would be the responsibility of the educated. The Jacksonian concept of democracy, however, with every man (and eventually woman, now, both from age 18 on) as a voter made the study of civics or government seem necessary, a beginning for functional subjects.

---

[11] Jefferson, Thomas in Letter to Col. Charles Yancy (Jan. 6, 1816) in Bartlett, John, *Familiar Quotations*. Boston: Little, Brown & Co., 1882. pg. 375.

HEALTH EDUCATION ENTERS. Health education gained its entree into the schools largely through the zeal and dedication of the Women's Christian Temperance Union (WCTU). This movement, which gained its greatest strength during the last half of the 19th century and the first several decades of the 20th century, had as its original motive better health and well-being for working men and families. However, the leadership of the movement came to feel that the use of alcoholic beverages was the prime deterrent to the well-being of all and thus arose the determination to rid the U.S.A. of all such intoxicants. Education of the young was obviously a necessity, and so, for the good of society, by 1890 every state in the U.S.A. had enacted legislation requiring instruction about the effects of (and in many instances the evils of) alcohol and narcotics. In 40 states, the laws specified that the instruction be part of a broader program of teaching physiology and hygiene.

THE "STAMP IT OUT" MOTIVE. Before going on, it is important to note the continuing significance of this beginning for health instruction in the schools. It came about because of the fervor of a special interest group, who wanted the school to help do something about the liquor problem. Still today, over 80 years later, the main impetus for instituting a health instruction program where one is not functioning is a desire to help do something about the drug problem . . . VD problem . . . accident problem . . . nutrition problem. . . . Even established programs may be called upon to produce evidence as to how they are doing on these currently relevant problems. What this seems to say is that health education has not generally been accepted as a legitimate part of general education, but must be continuously justified on the basis of preventing something undesirable from happening.

CHILD DEVELOPMENT MOTIVES. It would be inaccurate to characterize this concept of the school as a departure from the strictly intellectual institution as being motivated simply by societal needs. The child study movement, started in the 1890's by Stanley Hall, Felix Adler and William H. Burnham, among others, saw the school as a means to meet certain needs in individual youngsters that were being neglected by the non-school influences in their lives. Studies in child development illuminated physical, mental, emotional, and social needs; these had to be met where children were . . . and obviously they were in school for a significant part of their waking day for a good portion of the year. Perhaps the most accurate description, then, was that the schools were seen as social institutions responsible for dealing with the personal needs and problems of youngsters.

This view had its effect on educational philosophy, with its first obvious apogee being the Progressive Educational Movement with John Dewey's concept that learning was best when the whole child was actively involved in the process, including that of setting the goals for the learning experience.[12]

HEALTH AND PHYSICAL EDUCATION. At about the same time (the tail end of the 19th century), physical education programs were being devised and instituted in schools (enough children were no longer working hard physically and were becoming soft, sedentary creatures) as another problem-solver. Since a number of laws mentioned the teaching of health habits, many school administrators came to lump these utilitarian subjects together because of the apparent similarities between the two, and the phenomenon of health and physical education emerged. The generally unfortunate effects of this for health education will be expanded later in the volume.

GENERAL OR USEFUL? Today, among the many people interested in school health education, there is not likely to be agreement as to the institution of which it should be a part. Those who would prefer to see it as a part of general, liberal education envision the subject field as a medium by which learners can achieve a better more complete view of themselves, other people and the environment in which they live—somewhat comparable to studies of literature, American history, and geography. They would be minimally concerned as to exactly what the behaviors of learners were after health education, confident that the educated person makes the best decision.

At the other extreme (of a continuum, since there is no evidence that health education personnel fall neatly into two dichotomous camps) are folk who see health education as clearly utilitarian and functional, studied because certain behaviors are better for individuals and for society than other behaviors. They would be maximally concerned that health education produce definite desired behaviors and non-behaviors —i.e., eating of a balanced diet, non-smoking, exercising regularly, not having sexual relations with the venereally diseased, seeing an MD for a wide variety of symptoms, etc.

At the first extreme there is maximum faith in the rationality of the human being to do what he/she knows is best, and maximum faith that education, where all facts and viewpoints and values are considered, will produce the best behavior. At the other extreme, there is little faith that learners can translate ideas into the best behavior, maximum fear that real education will encourage them to do what they should not, and therefore maximum commitment to propaganda and conditioning, conscientiously pushing for a particular behavior or non-behavior as being the best for the individual and for society.

---

[12] ASCD 1972 Yearbook Committee, Squire, James R. (Ed.), *A New Look at Progressive Education*. Washington, D.C.: Association for Supervision and Curriculum Development, 1972. Introduction, pp. 1-13.

LIFE BETWEEN THE EXTREMES. Probably many, if not most, health educators are somewhere between these extremes. Some years ago I suggested, partly seriously (as an illustration of this eclectic modality) and partly in jest, that the actual goal of teachers in alcohol education should be stated as, "We help students to consider all the facts so that they can make up their own minds—not to drink." The day-to-day behavior of many teachers mirrors compromises like this one: they want students to deal with a variety of facts, ideas, concepts, and value systems, but they truly know what behavior decisions they want for their learners. Though they know that much learning about health-related behavior comes from actual experiences, they are reluctant to sanction experimental behaviors like drinking beer, smoking marijuana, overeating, or fighting . . . let alone ones like taking LSD, contracting venereal disease, or getting no treatment for a severe wound. A major raison d'être of school health education is that everyone does not have to learn by actual experience—many young people can learn many things vicariously . . . accepting the experience of others (particularly when systematically and scientifically analyzed) as evidence that some behaviors are likely to be desirable and others undesirable.

Okay, the generalization would be that though teachers of health will vary from the very permissive to the very directive, most will exhibit some desire for students to make their own decisions, conglomerated with some desire for students to avoid potential pain and harm.

THREE BASIC PHILOSOPHIES. This really suggests that health teachers tend to be eclectic in philosophy, and purist philosophers try to argue that every educator must have some basic assumptions about reality, knowledge, and how learning takes place . . . that one can't believe everything at the same time. Let's consider, but briefly, three relatively differentiated educational philosophies and what a health educator would assume if she/he embraced each.

The realist health educator assumes that knowledge exists as a real entity and therefore sees the task as using the most efficient means to bring learners and knowledge together.

The idealist (should really be ideaist, but this doesn't pronounce well) health educator assumes that knowledge exists in minds and therefore attempts to establish direct contact with the minds of learners in order to have them learn what she/he knows.

The experimentalist health educator assumes that knowledge is created anew in the mind of each learner and since this creation is an active process she/he devises ways for students to be actively involved in the learning process.

In short, the ways in which health educators go about their tasks are affected by their assumptions about knowledge and about how learning takes place. Each of these philosophies is back of some successful

... and some unsuccessful ... health education. None can be proven false, so it seems probable that diversity of approach to learning about health will continue.

PLEASE RECALL ... What should be emphasized for recall from this chapter? No new, sparkling, startling or cogent definition of health is offered; rather, the term is used to refer to the quality of functioning of a person in totality: How you are and what you did in the altogether. It can be seen as a state of being or as the process of functioning; it can be assessed as any moment, or it can be judged over some longer period of time.

- Though health is fundamentally the condition for functioning of an individual, some behaviors and some non-behaviors can be called healthy and others unhealthy on the basis of central tendencies in results. There probably are no behaviors that everyone agrees are absolutely healthy or unhealthy, but modern science and the much older pragmatic perception of people combine to give a basis for health education. Health education goes on continuously, because it can relate to any and all of the behaviors that make up an active day, week ... and, ultimately, life. Knowledge, attitudes, behavior ... or what you know, how you feel, and what you do and do not do, are constantly being reinforced, modified, changed—or some dynamic combination of these.

- Health education belongs in the schools. The answer to this affirmation is both Yes and No. It can be seen as part of general education, a medium for better understanding self and the rest of the world. It can be seen as a supreme example of practical study, learning ways of behaving that make life better, and learning to avoid those that carry a portent of harm. But unfortunately and realistically, it also can be seen as content of such personal and value-laden nature that the school should steer clear. And yet, if ignorance contributes to social upset, must the schools not be involved? And so it goes. ...

- Educational philosophy involves one's assumption about how learning takes place, and the three competing philosophies each suggest a different crucial element—the material to be learned, the teacher, or the activity of the learner.

- Health education is a discipline or arena of teaching-learning that focuses on motivation and communication. Learners must be motivated to learn and then communicated with in ways that keep their motivations from dwindling. For these reasons alone, it is a human activity that is both challenging and frustrating.

Chapter III

Health in the U.S.A. -Mid-1970's

What is your expectation for a chapter that would seem to be an overview of health in this country at about this time? One might expect biostatistics, detailing and charting death rates, disease rates, accident sites, causes of death by age groups . . . and so on. Another expectation might be a chronicling of evidence that we have made progress in health because children, youth, and adults do not die as early nor do they die of the same diseases and conditions. Each of these has merit, and other authors have written quite competently using these as bases. But how about an expectation that the generalizations which the statistics generate are perhaps more important than the numbers and that our present situation encourages some diverse philosophical positions? This probably is not the usual interpretation, but it should be the one the reader considers when reading the following pages.

THE CRITERION? HEALTH. Let's go back. Health, as described in the first portion of this book, is the quality of function—of living— of the total person. Dying of tuberculosis, typhoid, or smallpox at an early age certainly is not healthy, but simply not dying of these (or even contracting them) is not necessarily healthy either. It rather depends on what one is doing—or how one is living—when one is not having tuberculosis, typhoid, or smallpox. So, the status of health of people within American culture must be assessed at least as much in terms of how they are functioning as in terms of the past disease threats they are encountering or are overcoming. Such an assessment obviously involves more value judgments than are involved in comparing percentages and past cases with those of the present.

RELATIVE OR ABSOLUTE. Another interesting value judgment that is involved in assessing health status is that of the difference between what has been accomplished since . . . (sometime past) and what could have been or should have been accomplished. Is our health good because fewer people die of pneumonia than 50 years ago, or is it poor because some folks still die of this essentially preventable condition? Are we a well-nourished nation because the majority gets a better balance of nutrients in their diet than was true 50 years ago, or are we a poorly nourished nation because all do not enjoy this balance? Both sorts of judgments can be—and are—made. Each judgment is based on a different chosen criterion . . . and there is no scientific or agreed-upon way to select the right criterion.

HYGEIA AND ASCLEPIUS. Another important perspective for this discussion is one I shall borrow from the distinguished health philosopher, Rene Dubos. In his *Mirage of Health*[1] he developed the philosophic and practical differences between the mythological personages of Hygeia and Asclepius and between their ancient and modern-day followers. Dubos' scholarship tells us that the term "hygiene," often used for health education before the 1940's, comes from the cult of Hygeia, a lovely goddess who probably was a personification of Athena, the goddess of reason. Hygeia was not related to treatment of the sick, but, rather, was seen as the guardian of health and symbolized the belief that men could remain well if they lived according to reason. Hygeia stood for the virtue of a sane life in a pleasant environment, and, in Greece, was closely identified with mental health. According to Dubos (and important for health education efforts today), she never really "touched the hearts of the people." After the fifth century B.C., her influence became less than that of the healing god, Asclepius.

According to Greek legend, Asclepius was the first physician, a master in the use of the surgical knife and in the knowledge of curative plants. He was a handsome, self-assured young god, looked to by the increasing number of folk who were not willing to attempt the difficult task of living wisely.

Dubos sums up both the ancient and mythical and modern contemporary differences in view of health embodied in these two:[2]

> For the worshippers of Hygeia, health is the natural order of things, a positive attribute to which men are entitled IF they govern their lives wisely. According to them the most important function of medicine is to discover and teach the natural laws that will ensure to man a healthy mind in a healthy body. More skeptical and wiser in the ways of the world, the followers of Asclepius believe that the chief role of the physician is to treat disease, to restore health by correcting any imperfection caused by the accidents of birth or of life.

Hence, it is not just a phenomenon of modern life and times that progress and problems in health are perceived differently.

ADAPTATION. A later chapter will develop an ecological perspective for health, which seems to be an important one to understand, even if one cannot accept it as a major premise to live by. In a miniscule preview of that perspective, let's consider the concept of adaptation.

---

[1] Dubos, Rene, *Mirage of Health*, Garden City, New York: Doubleday & Co., Inc., Anchor Books, 1961, pp. 113-114.

[2] Ibid. By permission of Harper & Row.

Adapting to the environment is what is necessary for the effective survival (healthy functioning) of every form of life. People, as the highest form of life, in addition to adapting (1) can change the environment so that adaptation is easier and (2) can avail themselves of human-developed means to strengthen their capacity to adapt. They can (1) plant trees or put up other forms of shade to protect themselves from the sun; they can wear clothes and live in a heated house to help adapt to cold weather; they can take an antibiotic so that an infection will not develop further . . . and (2) they can be immunized against tetanus to prevent that disease; they can use a toothbrush, a fluoride toothpaste, and dental floss to retard and prevent tooth decay; they can wear glasses in order to read ordinary type after farsightedness has developed. . . . The point is not whether or not people should change their external and their internal environments (making adapting easier or unnecessary) but what the balance should be between the individual using her/his own individual resources and not having to adapt. Stanley, a hypothetical human (whose views might help now), leans toward adapting as much as possible by his own means on the premise that the more he has to adapt, the more ready he will be to adapt when truly necessary. A well-known old Greek physician, Hippocrates, discovered and uttered what he considered a great truth, which bulwarks Stanley's premise nicely. Stanley quotes him thus: "All parts of the body that are designed for a definite use are kept in health and in enjoyment of fair growth and of long youth by the fulfillment of that use and by their suitable exercise in the duty for which they were made."

However, many situations of adaptation have a risk involved; if the individual fails in the attempt to adapt, there will be some harm, pain, disablement, or even death. This leads to the opposite health-oriented admonition. Avoid risks whenever you can. A homey example: Our third son was not quite four years old, but he was watching with envy his two older brothers as they often walked the 2″ by 4″ board that capped the six foot fence that enclosed our back yard. This was some act of youthful daring, but it was also an adaptation: perfecting balance and foot-eye coordination, becoming comfortable in functioning off the ground . . . and also doing something some of their friends could not or would not attempt. One morning, as I watched from inside the house, this not-quite four year old, Ricky, all by himself, climbed to the top of the fence, sat there for awhile, then slowly and carefully got to his feet and took a couple of steps. Just about that time, the phone rang, signalling the anxious voice of the lady next door advising me to get Ricky down from the fence before he fell. It was a natural piece of advice, but as I listened to her I could also see the look of delightful, final accomplishment on his young face as he edged along the fence. In a few minutes he came down, and I congratulated him rather than admonishing him about the danger. There was a danger, of course, and I refused to visualize the consequences to that bright, young face should he have lost his balance and smashed his visage on the cement below. Which was the healthy behavior—learning to adapt to the high fence with the risk there, or staying off the fence 'cause you might fall? One can't really learn to adapt without adapting, and may not be able to practice adapting without risks. A total chapter will be devoted to this important and vexing health issue: "Risk-Taking."

HEALTH PERSONNEL. If any man or woman on the street were asked to identify some health personnel, the chances are whopping that he/she would name doctor or physician, then probably nurse . . . and it is doubtful that health educator would be included at all, without some coaching from the sidelines. Most Americans, then, would be Asclepians, associating health with doctoring. A consciousness of health is aroused in many people only when some condition or ill-health arises. The expectation then builds that health will return via the wise, skilled, and knowledgeable personal physician, who will diagnose accurately and treat promptly and properly. Each legitimate practitioner of the medical art presumably reveres and follows the oath of Hippocrates, who generally gets the credit for separating the practice of medicine from that of magic. The Hippocratic oath says:[3]

> I will follow that method of treatment which, according to my ability and judgment, I consider for the benefit of my patients, and abstain from whatever is deleterious and mischievous.

To sum up: "Health" is probably most often associated with "physician," and the physician is most often oriented to a method of treatment and the benefit of the sick.

A HIPPOCRATIC HEALTH EDUCATOR. An interesting point is that the Hippocratic admonitions could also apply to a wider view of health, where the practitioners in addition to physicians, dentists, hygienists, and aides doing patient education as part of a coordinated health care delivery system, also include health educators. Consider:

> I will follow those methods of prevention, substitution, treatment, cure, rehabilitation, and reorientation of life values which . . . I consider for the benefit of my patients and the larger community.

Remember, health is to be nurtured and maintained as well as recaptured and rebuilt after loss.

Though the individual, one-to-one, doctor-patient relationship will remain germinal to medical practice—and hence to medical care—

[3] Hippocrates, Oath of, *Colliers Encyclopedia*. New York: The Crowell Collier Publishing Company, 1965. Volume 12, pg. 138. ("There are several translations of the Hippocratic oath, all fundamentally the same, and this is one of them. . . .")

increasingly physicians are performing their scientific art in a variety of patterns such as group practice, community clinics, and in industrial and military settings, where they are part of functioning teams of professional and allied health personnel. The very existence of such plans has an educating effect. Predictably the public view of health will broaden as it is dealt with in these ways, which are beyond the merely not sick.

A NON-STATISTICAL TOUR. Let's be off on our projected non-statistical treatment of health statistics. One of the fundamental indices of health, presumably, is the death rate—from specific causes and, overall, crude and adjusted. We believe that all deaths must have some medically diagnosable cause, and that all deaths must be statistically accounted for. We rank in order causes of death, and any listing presumably must total 100 percent. Thus, the decrease in a particular cause of death might temporarily lower the total death statistic, but eventually would be translated into a statistical increase in another cause. For example, a predictable result of a major breakthrough in cancer prevention and treatment, which would lower cancer to perhaps the tenth instead of the second leading cause of death, would create a statistical increase in death from heart disease, stroke, circulatory failure, and accidents. It is generally assumed that death is bad and that post-poning death is good. Death control is an established good, with a basic ethic of the medical and nursing professions being the prolonga-tion of life. If we had a cause-of-death category labelled "old age" based on some agreed-upon acceptance of death as normative beyond a certain age, then we might truly make some progress in reducing death. But our present expectations simply can never be realized.

AS THE POPULATION GETS OLDER . . . Problems and frustra-tions about the health situation are likely to increase in the future also, because the prolongation of life in that certain-to-increase older portion of the American population will be increasingly costly in money and professional time and attention. Thus, what could be done will not be available for some, and because it should be, our society's health will be judged inferior. Dubos,[4] again, raised the value question, para-phrased as: Is a culture healthier when it spends an increasing amount of its resources on health maintenance and death avoidance? Would the ultimate healthy society be one in which half the population were therapists, of one type or another, for the other half? Or would this be the ultimate absurd distortion of a truly humane goal?

I admitted at the beginning that figures can be helpful in making a generalization, so I do not consider the following hypocritical. 1972

---

[4] Dubos, Rene, *The Dreams of Reason, Science and Utopias,* New York: Columbia University Press, 1961. pp. 82-96.

statistics showed that the aging (over 65) comprised one tenth of the population but were responsible for over one quarter of the total health spending. This differential between the services for young and old is often interpreted to mean that the young, healthy, and productive are paying the bills for the older, unemployed infirm. The fact is, however, that the majority of older citizens pay their own way through savings, investments, etc. Many use social security benefits into which they have paid their fair share during their years of employment.

MENTAL HEALTH. To symbolize a broader view of health, let us postpone the chronicling of physical gains and losses and begin with mental and social (and possible spiritual) dimensions of well-being. In the mental realm, the population has considerable structured education, and through this and other formal means and mass media, has more knowledge relative to our past and to most other cultures today. Paradoxically, because knowledge is increasing beyond our capacity to absorb it, in relation to what there is to know, we become relatively more ignorant each year. Are we more or less healthy in terms of knowing? Pick your criterion. Youth, particularly, seem to be more curious and more experimental. These characteristics encourage change . . . of many kinds, some clearly laudible, some clearly dangerous, and some not clearly. . . .

In the young and not-still-young population there seems to be more searching for self. Is this a healthy development? For those who gain some previously lacking self-perception and translate this into happy, positive functioning, the trend seems healthy. But some seek more self than they are able to find without some more living; the less healthy paths from this dilemma seem to lead to more frantic, bizarre searching instead of more balanced living or a lethargic hopelessness . . . "Here I am nineteen and I haven't discovered who I really am! (sob!)" Expectations about "having one's head on straight" seem to be high, which in one sense is commendable and in another almost assures that there will be frustrations and consequent lack of comfortable, positive living. Again the value question: are we a healthier nation because greater numbers of people are seeking some kind of help with emotional problems and personality functioning? Or are there increasing numbers of Americans who simply cannot cope with the complexities of the culture?

SOCIAL-CULTURAL. This question eases us into the social-cultural realm and the relative status of healthy relationships of people, one with another, groups with other groups, and people and groups with societal institutions. The positive analysis is that societal health is good and constantly improving because there is increasing freedom for individuals and groups to function in nonstereotypic ways. Relationships between people are less firmly established and set than in times past, so those relationships that develop are more conscious and potentially more genuine and require some maintenance, rather than being automatic and enduring because there are no viable alternatives. Most people are freer to move from group to group and there is a definite diminishing of any established caste and class system. Strong forces for equality of opportunity for females in a traditionally male-dominant culture are rather rapidly being translated into action, laws, and new mores.

However, again, we are far from our expectations and the ideal society. Freedom of relationships means some folk succeed . . . but others do not or are not able to develop satisfying relations. People, groups, and institutions compete, and animosities develop and are expressed. Stability is hard to come by, and those who cannot adapt to mobility and change can be very unhappy and sadly dysfunctional. The freedom that the majority has is not shared by minorities—the lower class, the handicapped, the non-whites and others. New mores and practices relative to equality of male and female can further fractionate the society and fan the fires of resentment, bitterness, and social upset. A society probably cannot change, particularly in several directions and dimensions at the same time and within a relatively short time, without some amount of social turmoil. Is this a sign of social health—that we are going through a period of disequilibrium in order to accomplish some worthwhile changes? The evaluation can be—and is—made both ways.

An analogy from the physical realm: An overweight person may have to experience some traumatic times in dieting to lose the protuberant poundage, but the final result may be more physically healthy, emotionally satisfying, and socially applauded. Yet, if she/he seeks to lose too much too rapidly or submits to questionable therapies even though the goal is a worthy one, the means may put more stress on the body than the original obesity. The solution to the problem may be worse than the problem. But in the social realm, no one can seem to make it perfectly clear whether the results of present changes in mores and practices will be for society's benefit or whether it can survive the process.

LIFE AND DEATH. Okay, speaking of deaths, let's look at our progress and problems in this more traditional manner of measuring health . . . in our now-established minimum statistical modality. The general trend and situation is that deaths are down and births are up and going down again. To clarify: the number of people actually dying when compared with the total population (all of whom could possibly die) is low in comparison to that of the earth's total human population. It is lower than in any previous period in American history. However, it is not as low as in some smaller, more homogeneous European countries, and certainly not as low as it theoretically could be . . . or should be. Births increased after World War II and were relatively high (meaning that more children were born and lived than necessary to replace the two biological parents) for many of the next twenty-five years. The last few years have been marked by reduction in both numbers and rate of births, and though it may be early to judge, society is beginning to consider this a fairly definite trend. Overall, however, the U.S. population is still increasing, and a stabilized number of citizens is unlikely before the commencement of the next century.

Length of life, the positive attribute to the death rate statistics, is obviously not uniform for all those born, and is not even uniform in averages for sub-groups in the population. Females live about seven and a half years longer than males, on the average. Whites live longer than non-whites or non-Anglos; middle to upper income people live longer than those with lower incomes. Thus, though the chances for longer life are relatively good if one is born an American, there are, on the average, better chances in being a white female in an upper-middle class home than in being a black male born and raised in a low income inner city neighborhood.

There has been relatively little actual lengthening of life in the last half-century. There always have been very old people—those in their 80's, 90's, and a few beyond, and there still are, but we can measure no significant relative increase in the numbers of those reaching these ages beyond the statistical average. As the infant and child mortality of our early years and the past century has been dramatically decreased through improved and more available medical facilities and through drugs to control infections, the statistical length of life has increased. But the principal killers of older people—heart and circulatory diseases and cancer—still afflict a majority of the past-the-prime population, so at present it is still comparatively unlikely that most individuals will live more than ten or fifteen years beyond retirement.

MICROORGANISMS NOT CONQUERED. No . . . even though the aforementioned reductions in mortality indicate that infectious diseases and conditions have been relatively controlled by immunizations, antibiotics and prompt knowledge-based care, they have not been eliminated. They have only been curbed from causing the deaths they once did. However, our controls work best when microorganisms act predictably, and even our scientists have relatively little control over the microorganism's capacity to mutate. So as long as germs are reasonably lethargic about mutating, we will maintain the upper hand. But should this not prevail, humans will have to scurry to adapt to the new threats—for an increasingly large and vulnerable population.

Another potential chink in our armor against infectious diseases is the lack of continuous concern for maintaining immunization levels at all age levels. Many small babies are immunized against diphtheria, whooping cough (pertussis), measles, mumps, poliomyelitis and rubella. Schools frequently require booster immunizations at certain points, but after this, except for young people entering the military service, society has no way of compelling people to keep their immunities high. It is possible, then, that without these diseases present in the population in hidden, sub-clinical form, the vulnerability of the populace—or parts of it—may be increasing. This would probably not be known until there was an actual outbreak of, say, diphtheria.

Another interesting development with some potential for reducing national immunities is that during the 1960's vital statistics indicated that there were no cases of smallpox, but a fairly predictable dozen or so deaths per year attributable to the vaccination. One possible judgment would have been that these constitute an acceptably low number of deaths, the cost of maintaining protection against an awful, killing, and disfiguring disease. But the obviousness of the original threat has faded, and the value that has prevailed is that society should not require a procedure that has even this risk factor. So required smallpox reimmunizations for school attendance are disappearing, and unless parents accept the personal responsibility for making sure their children's immunity is satisfactory the portion of the population vulnerable to the disease smallpox will rise. In summary, our control of infectious diseases and conditions is quite commendable (though far from perfect) and should stay this way and improve if the life forms in the microscopic world stay relatively constant and predictable. And over this we have little control.

IS LARGER HEALTHIER? Reduction in incidence of certain diseases is an indication of health progress; are there other physical measures? The Fifth Edition of this book took the logical position that reduced infections, better nutrition, and better living conditions made for better physical health, which resulted in increased weight and height averages for American children. It is often assumed that continued growth automatically equates with better health. However, there is no clear, agreed-upon, proven ideal size for children, youth, or adults, and so perhaps we have acceded to the good ol' American standard of the bigger, the better. There is little doubt that a good seven foot basketball center is better than the typical six foot three tip-off man of a quarter century back and the two hundred sixty pound pro lineman is more effective than his counterpart at two hundred ten pounds. But as our population increases and then agglomerates in urban areas, will larger size make for better functioning? Driving smaller automobiles would conserve gasoline. Will increasing size be a healthy trend? The typical U.S. youngster enjoys one of the best protein-rich diets in the world, with whole milk, eggs, beef, and pork as main sources of complete amino-acid building blocks. Yet these also may start typical Dick and Jane Americans off with regular high saturated fat diets, which some medical scientists feel encourage the build-up in cholesterol in the circulatory system. Eating patterns established in childhood and youth, based on a minimum of three balanced meals each day plus socially valuable snack times, if not changed when the person becomes a more sedentary adult, can result in overnutrition with resulting obesity, which may impede full functioning in the physical, social, and mental dimensions.

IS ADAPTATION HEALTHY? Thus, nutritional scientists observed the undesirable effects of certain deficiencies and then determined logically and empirically that providing the deficient nutrient would and did correct the deficiency and thus make for better health. This correcting-the-deficiency modality obviously was beneficial because without the deficiency the patient functioned more fully in the observable now. But Dubos suggests both an intriguing and a disturbing contraindication. The developmental history of human beings, from a nutritional perspective, has largely been one of feast and famine, with irregularities and cyclical changes in food available. Each early human obviously had to develop the adaptive mechanisms for this situation if he/she was to survive. Dubos says, "It may turn out that a nutritional way of living permitting continuous growth at a maximum rate may have unfortunate distant results . . . [by not] providing an opportunity for the operation of certain emergency mechanisms built by nature into the human body."[5] If the body does not have to adapt, it may not develop the mechanism to do so. Thus, it is possible that civilized people could see their analogue in the laboratory animal raised in a germ free environment. It grows beautifully and functions well within its environment, but cannot survive and function well outside. Then, in a true scientific sense we and our children are part of an experiment. The hypothesis we are testing is that regular, balanced meals leading to maximum growth will produce healthy human beings who can function well in all kinds of situations. Obviously this test must run over sometime and encompass many situations, including natural ones in which the expected good is not present. Our hypothesis still seems a good one; we just must not claim, with too much dogmatism, the superiority of bigger is better.

DEATH AS PROBLEM. Quite obviously my treatment of our health progress did not include a clear differentiation from our problems. In a real sense some of our progress sows the seed for new problems, and our problems provide the challenge for real progress.

[5] Dubos, Rene, *Mirage of Health.* pg. 155.

As already indicated, the public and the medical profession in general tend to see the number one problem as the various causes of death. Progress in solving this problem—i.e., postponing death and prolonging life—seems generally commendable. This, however, presents us with the increasing problem of maintaining the desired reverence and respect for and value upon human life. If the focus is on the young, as health education in the school typically is, then the number one problem is not so much sidestepping threats to one's existence and thereby avoiding death. It isn't even a problem, really; it is the challenge of living life as fully as possible in the midst of threats to its quality.

However, let us look at the reasons for death, their causes and possible solutions. As already chronicled, accidents are the major cause of the early demise of children and youth. The basic reasons for this phenomenon can be differentiated as (1) the relatively large numbers of the young (2) the complexity of the culture, where learning safe behavior is not only time-consuming but virtually continuous (3) the appeals of risk-taking behavior over safer behavior and (4) chance—or the fact that things just do not always happen the way they should or usually do. If there are reasons for accidents, then reduction of this mortality category would hinge on these being changed. The chances? Well, the numbers of youth are being reduced, but the general trend seems to be to more complexity in the culture rather than less. Perhaps there are ways to condition children more completely toward safe rather than risky behavior, but it does not seem clear that we want to take the risk of using them universally. Since chance is a factor over which, by definition, we have little control, there seem to be no evident ways to make the world utterly predictable. So, we would affect some reduction in numbers and even rate of accidents,but, barring some unforeseen snatcher of lives (e.g., radiation, some mutated microorganism), accidents seem certain to remain number one. Mostly, remember, because there are no real competitors for the lives of our basically healthy young people.

Death from malignancies could be reduced when medical science discovers the reason or reasons why deranged and disorderly cells begin to grow. If there are factors that start a cancer, can these be prevented or effectively destroyed in early stages? If normal body factors that prevent development of malignancies in most individuals are missing or deficient in a relative few, can these factors be stimulated or provided? So, basic discovery and subsequent translation into practical prevention and treatment are the first requisites; then relative success would hinge on the comprehensiveness of the health and medical care delivery system (including health education) and the priority evolved for the young.

Deaths from congenital malformations and forms of heart disease reflect a generally poor capacity to adapt to the world and its various potential threats. A perspective to set quickly is that many children and youth with congenital malformations and heart disease do survive; some live relatively normally, others live with difficulty (often sustained by some super-desire to be a part of this world's human community), and others barely survive, often kept alive by complex medical technology. Improvement in mortality rates, then, would come from more discovery and implementation and perhaps from the yet relatively speculative field of biological engineering. Creative tampering within this field might prevent certain predictable anomalies. Yet, again, real success would come only with their availability to all of the population.

Homicide and suicide, two growing reasons for youth death, can be catalogued on a sociological matrix pointing to the many ways in which the society does not allow all children and youth to develop positive attitudes and their full potential. An eclectic combination leads to the broad generalization that some of the young have spells of genuinely poor personal adaptation to the culture. Translated, this can mean that the culture makes it possible for a youth to possess a loaded handgun; in certain ways it encourages animosities between groups; and it still indicates there is a good in defending the honor of one's family, friends, or group. So, when Sam calls Johnny Bob's sister a name reflecting on her virtue, Johnny Bob can get angry enough with Sam and what he represents to shoot him and kill him. Objectively, this is poor adaptation on both of their parts and should be prevented. But, again, there are many ways to prevent other destructive or self-destructive behavior . . . that work with the big majority. We simply are not able or willing to try for perfection.

ABUSE OF MOOD MODIFYING SUBSTANCES. To reiterate the general philosophy of this chapter: the health problems of children and youth are not so much those that kill as those that reduce present functioning and that abort growth and development so that future functioning as an adult is seriously jeopardized. Some examples of such that are prominent in the first portion of the 1970's are abuse of substances that modify mood and behavior (alcohol and other forms of drug substances), venereal disease, and several forms of mental illness. Of course, there are also some deaths due to driving while intoxicated, to heroin and barbiturate overdoses, and to bizarre behavior while on some other drug trip. However, the effects on behavior (short of death) are more reason for educational concern at this time. The perspective, which may be becoming a familiar one, is that the majority of young people do not abuse themselves with alcohol or with drugs; some of these do not use mood and behavior modifying substances at all, and others use them infrequently.

Of course, the substances are available in a wide range of forms, they do chemically change the mind functioning, and changes from normal are often harmful. The greatest potential health hazard, how-ever, is that young abusers may not learn other, more useful (and often more difficult) forms of adjustment to life circumstances and thus are unprepared to live and function as adults without chemical crutches. It is thus an interesting value question whether it is healthier for a young abuser to survive all threats to life and then live a long life as a personally miserable human, inflicting misery and expense on others, and contributing little or nothing to the life of others or to society.

VENEREAL DISEASE. VD is another recognized health problem of youth. It will be argued by some that VD is the problem, while others counter that VD is only a result of the problem of promiscuous sexual intercourse, heterosexual and homosexual. In classic disease analysis, the main effect is slow deterioration of body tissues and organs, resulting in premature death. Gonorrhea has two more immediate results, which would qualify it as a youth health problem—pain (in the male, mainly), which can reduce normal functioning, and potential sterility, eliminating the possibility of being a biological parent. The venereal diseases, how-ever, deserve more than the label of mental and social problems. Our general social values equate contracting VD with being outside the mores of the culture that encourages feelings of shame, guilt, and anxiety. Receiving a case of syphilis from a friend is considered far from the ideal Valentine's Day gift, and the passing on of same tends to provoke emotional and social upset. Thus, the ultimate problem may be one of a lack of responsibility—a lack of feeling and concern for others, when this may interfere with one's own pleasure.

Concepts of mental ill-health continue to evolve, with more viable and practiced forms of treatment and prevention than in years past. Classic forms of schizophrenia, for example, continue to occur in a few instances, but the health problems are more abundant in the larger numbers of young Americans who have much less sense of self-identity than they aspire to have, who exhibit purposelessness and an often frightening degree of anomie, who lack the desire for association with other persons and with institutions, and who suffer from paralyzing spells of depression. These departures from health obviously have some ring-around-the-rosy relationship to alcohol and drug abuse, sexual promiscuity, homicide, suicide, and accidents. Discussion of each will be expanded later in conjunction with the health educational challenges unique to each and common to all.

One other problem of youth often discussed in term of lamentation is DENTAL ILL-HEALTH. This includes tooth decay, broken teeth, poor tooth alignment, illness of the oral cavity, and their effects on general health. It is true that the knowledge and skill to repair and even prevent oral problems has increased tremendously in the last few decades, but is available to only a limited portion of the population.

We probably do as much educating for good mouth care as for **any** other aspect of health in the elementary years. But most of the good practices (mainly brushing and flossing the teeth a time or two each day) are about neutralized or overcome by such factors as our civilized diet. Repair is necessary for most persons. People seldom die of dental problems so they have not the urgency of less widespread but potentially more fatal conditions. There are barely enough dentists to take care of present demands, and, except for emergencies, even conscientious people often must wait months for appointments. As supply does increase, demand rises even beyond. We have an able and dedicated professional cadre of dentists, hygienists, and technicians, who do miraculous work on individual mouths, but fall ever behind in being able to do much for all. And we, the society, sort of accept this as one of our endemic problems. It is increasingly clear that prevention through self-care is the only possible solution at this time.

FULLER FUNCTIONING. Finally, the goal of pre-professionals and professionals, at any and all levels, perusing this book is to encourage better health or fuller capacity to function as human beings, perhaps more specifically for Americans and particularly for children and youth. In some ways the culture is making progress toward this goal. In other ways, we seem to be creating new problems or threats to health. For example, within the last several decades we have experienced the development and accessibility of both penicillin and DDT. In yet other ways, our progress—our solutions—directly creates new problems, which then necessitates deciding what we can tolerate and what problems must be (at least partially) resolved. Health education deals with both treatment and prevention. Prevention is the greater challenge, but is the more difficult to demonstrate. Health education deals with facts and with valuing. Dealing with valuing is the greater challenge, yet it is more difficult to evaluate. For what is success? It certainly is not just getting students to accept the educator's personal values (though these may be quite desirable). But the task of evaluating any exercise in value classification is a value dilemma in itself. One class explores the values involved in marijuana legislation; about half accepts society's right to protect itself against free use of another mood modifier, while the other half values the right of the individual to decide whether she/he will or will not use such a substance. All simply do not see its potential danger in the same way. Another class tries to clarify the values involved in death; about 60 percent come to feel that after a certain age, say 70 years, death should be considered natural and no attempts made to prolong life; the other students value life more and feel each life should be maintained as long as possible. Is one value better than another? Or can the teacher be satisfied and have the faith that the process of valuing is the important item to be learned?

A SUMMARY

- Status of health is more a matter of how well people are functioning than merely not dying of certain conditions.
- Health results from some balance between positive living (prevention) and proper, appropriate treatment and cure of illness and disability.
- Adaptation is a necessity for health, and young Americans must adapt to a variety of threats, including those mental and social.
- As the U.S. population increases in average age there will be need for more medical care; it has not yet been determined how such will be provided.
- The effects of infectious diseases are not as evident as in times past, but levels of immunity must be kept high.
- Larger bodies may not mean healthier humans.
- Causes of accidents, suicide, venereal disease, drug abuse, and many emotional disturbances are known, but the culture seems unwilling to take the steps that could eliminate them.

Medical education does not fold up because all patients do not recover and live forever. General education does not fade away because what is learned is not remembered and utilized. So health education should not fret and fume because all people do not live healthfully. We have made progress. There is still more to be made. What we do may make some differences. Doesn't this possibility deserve our best?

Chapter IV

The Nature
of
the Learners

"Lee is just like her father . . . she understands what she reads but is slow, slow. . . ."

"I notice a great difference in Tim this year, particularly in his ability to control his temper."

"I wish Geraldine were more interested in boys; I guess she's normal enough, but I certainly was interested at her age!"

"My son Jonathan handles the ball well and is developing a consistent shot . . . he's going to be a good basketball player when he gets to high school."

"Karen certainly gets depressed and moody when she has her period . . . I didn't think that happened anymore."

"Remember when Reggie was a wild, black militant . . . now he's studying hard to get to college and medical school."

"Gus and Helen seem young, but they say they've really considered everything carefully and definitely are in love and want to get married."

When health education takes place, there is a learner(s), something to be learned (knowledge, attitude, process, behavior), and a learning environment. In the school setting for health instruction (a type of more formalized, planned, and predictable education), there is typically a group of learners or a class and a teacher and possibly other learning facilitators. This chapter will focus on the nature of the first listed essential—the learners. The vital questions to be probed are: What are learners like? and Which of their characteristics most affect their learning?

The descriptive comments above are representative of some of these characteristics in learners. It would be a reasonable, orthodox approach to this task to say some things first about little children, then bigger pre-adolescent children, and, finally, adolescents. This type of analysis you have read before; so how about using the School Health Education Study's three Key Concepts[1] as the basic frame of reference.

THREE KEYS. . . . According to the School Health Education Study's thinking, all health education should help develop these three Key

[1] School Health Education Study Writing Group, *Health Education. A Conceptual Approach to Curriculum Design.* St. Paul: 3M Education Press, 1967. pg. 16.

Concepts, which are the big-picture living processes underlying the health of the individual.

- Growing and Developing is the on-going process that begins with conception and concludes with death, a process that strongly influences the basic, predictable ways in which an individual behaves.
- Interacting is the process by which the individual relates actively to her/his environment in situations, more or less unconsciously.
- Decision-making is the process of consciously choosing to act one way rather than another . . . to do something . . . or not do something.

These concepts interrelate comparably to the dimensions described in Chapter II; there is no necessary order or set relationships. Out of a situation of interacting, a person makes a decision, definitely influenced by how she/he has grown and developed to that point. The decision brings further situations of interacting, perhaps more decisions . . . and all of this influences the growing and developing process, as it is influenced by past growing and developing. Each concept, because it is a process underlying health, has all of the dimensions—physical, emotional, mental, social . . . and perhaps spiritual and aesthetic. But let's try the personal rather than the abstract.

THREE CONCEPTS IN HUMAN LIVING. By the time they are ready for school, Matt and Lucy each have interacted with their parents enough to know some things about marriage. Each has grown and developed as a child in the family of a married couple and is aware of some ways husband and wife relate to each other. Lucy and Matt interact with each other occasionally as they progress through school. At one point their interacting is described, by Matt, as the verse of a song.[2]

> I know that Lucy Higgins still loves me
> 'Cause she hit me with her lunch pail
> When I kicked her on the knee

They each grow and develop into puberty and occasionally interact by dating. Both decide they would like to go with each other seriously and so begin to interact in a more purposeful fashion. They begin to grow and develop as a couple, doing an increasing number of things together and discovering more and more about each other. They each graduate from high school, make some career decisions and enter into some learning-to-work training. Their personal relationship has grown into one of mutual attraction and love. They make many decisions about their sexual interacting. They also feel it is wise to postpone marriage for awhile. They continue to grow and develop as a loving

2 From "Go Tell Roger" by John Stewart and Randy Cierly. © 1965 Irving Music Inc. (BMI). All rights reserved. Used by permission.

couple, and, with the approval of their parents and friends, finally make the decision to marry. Their growing and developing continues . . . as they begin the next generation reenactment of marriage.

NOW, ONE BY ONE. Having portrayed these three Key Concepts in their natural interrelating existence, let's now use them one by one, as the framework for illuminating the nature of young learners.

"Each human being grows and develops in some ways like all other humans, in some ways like some others, and in some ways like no other creature."[3] It should be obvious that a teacher recognizes that all students in a class have not grown and developed in a like way or at the same rate. At the same time, without being able to assume some commonalities, a teacher could do nothing with a class—and education would have to consist of one adult teaching one child.

Schools developed out of a complexity of reasons, but two that are pertinent here are:

(1) As knowledge increased and life became somewhat more complex, cultures realized that all adults did not know enough about everything to adequately teach a child what she/he should know, so teaching became a vocation.

(2) As adults began to concentrate on vocations (baking, blacksmithing, trading, tailoring), they began to favor the development of schools so that less total adult time was spent teaching. Even though teaching a class of youngsters of even fairly like ignorance is inefficient compared to individual teaching, it is less frustrating for the majority of non-teaching adults. In summary, maximum learning for all does not occur in schools because growing and developing is not identical for each youngster. However, schools can point to some accomplishments because there is some predictable comparability in growing and developing.

Children and youth grow and develop in their capacity to perceive phenomena, to differentiate between such, and to generalize from what they experience. A general example: A first grader may know that beer is one of the things that some adults drink; a fifth grader may know that beer is an alcoholic beverage, related to, but milder than, wine, whiskey and other bottled goods sold in liquor stores; a tenth grader may know what beer tastes like and what its possible effects are; a twelfth grader may know a variety of brands and when and where beer drinking is and is not appropriate . . . and why. This growing and developing obviously can proceed at different rates for different kids, but it still is a process with some general predictability.

Youngsters grow and develop in their capacities to remember, memorize, reason, and finally, develop concepts—summaries of experi-

---

[3] School Health Education Study Writing Group, *Health Education.* pg. 16.

ences that give order to perceptions and help to guide behavior. These capacities derive from some unquantifiable admixture of hereditary and environmental factors. The most general assumption is that heredity determines some ceiling on performance (on, say memorizing), and the environment pushes one toward or holds one back from achieving this theoretical capacity. Intelligence and aptitude tests are designed to measure this inherent capacity, but since these cannot be administered until after a goodly amount of environmental influence, there is no total agreement that any test can show clearly a person's hereditary potential. The majority of relatively traditional schools assume fairly regular mental growth and development as a norm for all students. "By the end of fourth grade, Charlie and Susie and Slats and . . . should have achieved this . . . and . . . this . . . or she/he flunks. And flunking is not a good thing to do." The fact that the process is not as uniform as the school assumes is one basis for difficulty students have in school. Some are not able to keep up, while others are bored and bitter over the time spent on something they already have learned and know.

Another phenomenon exceedingly important to learning is attention span, also presumed to increase gradually and steadily as maturation takes place. Without attention the teacher can direct no predictable learning, and only as learners can keep their attention on the idea or process can they learn it well. Part of this growing and developing process is mental (capacity to direct and control the mind) and part is emotional (capacity to control emotions so that they do not interfere with this focusing of the intellect). Students almost always have less attention span than the teacher, but the teacher may persist with a point anyway. Various forms of reward and punishment are devised and utilized to increase attention span. Like, "This will be the focus of the most important question on Friday's test!" or, "Who would like to find a film that explains this idea for the class?" or some other positive thing.

Growing and development in the emotional dimension of being is certainly not an even, steady process for each lad and lass. Still, the general ability being developed is that of expressing and controlling emotions and feelings—learning to express feelings that need to be outwardly evidenced and to inhibit those that hamper good relations with teachers and other learners. The school, because it has to function as a social institution, too often may seem more interested in the young learner's control of emotions such as anger, jealousy, greed, and selfishness than in expressing feelings of gratitude, love, and desire to share. It is gratifying to know that there are schools that place as much emphasis on the latter characteristics as the former.

As with academic achievement, the school tends to expect fairly steady and predictable movement toward maturity in emotional expression. When this expectation is not met, the deviant may be beginning to grow and develop as a troublemaker (in his/her own eyes as well as those of the school) . . . or as an isolate not able to enter into interactions as expected.

One interesting predictable—and yet unpredictable—stage in emotional growing and developing comes in adolescence when it is fairly normal for them to act inconsistently. One day Melody may be very touchy and overreact, particularly to requests made of her. The next day she may underrract, seeming to be exceedingly lethargic and non-interested. During this period, teachers or parents cannot assume that the way Patrick responds is the way Patrick really feels. He may seem hyper-interested one day and volunteer to do all kinds of things . . . and never do them. Another time he may seem very uninterested, but some later evaluation shows he really was interested and learned . . . but didn't appear to even be there. Experimentation may be part of this . . . the need to really try something that all reason and good sense suggests is dangerous. Thus, for some youngsters, the message that drug use, for example, is dangerous, may be, in effect, an heraldic challenge to see for themselves. It is important for adults to realize this possible place in development and not expect complete rational adult responses. Nor should they be too quick to react to adolescent responses as if they were inappropriate adult behaviors.

Other characteristics, with some elements of both the mental and the emotional that schools, teachers and parents assume will develop steadily and noticeably are self-discipline, the ability to carry out tasks to completion in the time allotted (despite frustrations), and self-direction, the capacity to function well without direct and constant adult supervision. Youngsters in whom these characteristics develop early or as expected tend to be good students, active in other school affairs, and able to participate in out-of-school activities as well. Those who are self-disciplined and self-directed tend to be the leaders of most groups.

Perhaps the most general and important growing and developing is in the concept of and the acceptance of self as a unique, individual human being. This obviously begins to show early in life, before school, in a child knowing her/his name and responding to it . . . in claiming some things as hers/his . . . etc. Schools encourage this trend by requiring each student to "Put your name on your paper" and "Do your own work". . . even defining cheating, a behavior defined as undesirable, as presenting someone else's answer as your own. It is interesting to note that this definition is merely a cultural choice; in a more communally-oriented culture cheating could be defined as "putting down an individualistic answer you have not shared with the group."

GOAL-INTERDEPENDENCE. Our culture, then, encourages each young citizen to grow and develop as an individual—to move away from dependence on and identification with others into a state of independence. The achievement of this is not considered an end in itself. From a perspective of health, the attaining of independence allows one to comfortably move on into a state of interdependence that is an admixture of being independent self, having others dependent on you, and being voluntarily dependent on others.

Schools generally assume that this development goes on at a somewhat uniform rate, as evidenced by teacher statements such as, "Most of my fifth graders couldn't carry through that independent a project" . . ."Most of my eighth graders could do a project that independently, but I would have to give them continuing guidance" . . . "Most of my twelfth graders can devise, organize, and carry out that independent a project, with almost no supervision from me." This last statement may not represent the average teacher. Some teachers do hang on to the notion that students must be dependent on them. They do not really encourage the kind of independent learning that the final grade levels of required schooling should feature . . . as a transition to non-school life where independence in learning is a necessity. Of course, the posture probably is a good one for students going to college, where the general environment in relation to learning in the freshman year is still one of considerable dependence—required courses and doing well on teacher-constructed and -graded examinations. So despite some assumption of uniform development, it is obvious from observation that there is no specified time that all young Americans become independent and then interdependent. We have a heterogeneous culture with many forces and counter-forces. Individuals respond differently to the forces. Some find independence easy and invigorating; others see no particular merit in it; still other find it frightening and unattractive.

Thus, young people are pulled toward the state of mind emblazoned on a contemporary wall poster, which says,

> I do my thing, and you do your thing.
> I am not in this world to live up to your expectations.
> And you are not in this world to live up to mine.
> You are you and I am I.
> And if by chance we find each other, it's beautiful.
> If not, it can't be helped.[4]

I would add a line, "If not . . . it can't be helped." At the same time this hyper-individuality is challenged by social interacting that encourages the interdependence encapsulated in John Donne's words:[5]

> No man is an island entire of itself; every man is a piece of the
>   continent, a part of the main;
> If a clod be washed away by the sea, Europe is the less as if a
>   promontory were, as well as if a manor of thy

---

[4] © Real People Press 1969. All rights reserved.

[5] Donne, John, *Devotions XVII* in Bartlett, John, *Familiar Quotations*. Boston: Little, Brown & Co., 1955. pg. 218.

Friends or of thine own were; any man's death diminishes Me
    because I am involved in mankind; and therefore never
Send to know for whom the bell tolls; it tolls for thee.

The ideal healthy human, in our terms, is one who is able and likes to function independently, but also is able and likes to be part of a group.

PEER GROUPS. Peer groups begin to form even before school attendance, but the school setting encourages both formal and informal, productive and relatively nonproductive groupings. In many schools, then, the child learns that his identity is not just Kevin S., and that, in the future, his own personal number is 275-66-5477. He also learns that he is a student at Fred Hein School in Ms. Appleby's second-grade class. He also learns that he is in the Yellow Bird reading group, rides on bus No. 17, and may be in a group of boys who go to a movie on Saturday afternoon. He may also belong to another group in which hair is worn long enough to be over the ears.

Youngsters grow and develop, then, as members of groups, some of which are not consistent in their expectations for members. Part of successful growth and development is the capacity to function in groups that are increasingly structured and task-oriented. Some children in pre-adolescence, go through a stage of being in a neighborhood club or gang, before more organized forms at schools or in the community beckon. Perhaps in illustration of the flexibility or alternative-orientation of our culture, the rules in one such clubhouse included the following:

    9. Do not turn on the hose.
  10. If you turn on the hose, be sure and turn it off again.

Another part of successful adaptation is being a good, functioning member of several perhaps incongruous groups at the same time. As I think back to my high school days, I find myself functioning as the son in a small family, as a member of athletic teams, as a member of a rather non-scholastically oriented fraternity, as a member of such intellectual enterprises as the Writer's Club, Bohemian Club, Honor Society, and a church youth group. Most of these were unrelated to each other much of the time, so I tended to function somewhat differently in each one. Perhaps this was necessary preparation for adult life. In a fit of frustration some years back, I identified at least thirteen different roles I was currently playing, many of which were not only incongruous but competitive—like being a writer and being a husband . . . and a father. Or, perhaps, it was only because I had grown and developed as I did through the teens that I am able to balance the many disparate grabs for my time, attention, and commitment.

THE GROWTH AND DEVELOPMENT THAT HURTS. Naturally, all of growing and developing is not positive or neutral. Most young people who grow and develop as drug users and abusers, for example, also grow and develop as members of a group that is using drugs. The most difficult use pattern to change then, becomes one in which (1) the social group associations are positive and pleasant (or perhaps there are no real alternatives), (2) the user knows what he/she is doing and feels no shame or regret about it, (3) the physical effects are generally desirable and not often painful and (4) the experience seems often to be an uplifting one aesthetically and spiritually. This is total hookedness. For the individual to begin to grow and develop as a non-user (or at least as a non-abuser), there must be some change in reinforcement patterns, and the dimension most vulnerable to outside influence often is the social influence of others. Synanon initiated the model for effective rehabilitation from drug abuse with the live-in facility. Their ethic was that anyone who was "heavy into drugs" probably had no personality structure worth saving. Therefore, the group united in its desire to give up drugs could help one another, through often vicious confrontations in the synanon group sessions, to develop new, functional personalities. Group reinforcement of non-use and of new ways of thinking is as necessary as it was when the person was drug-using.

COMFORTABLE IN GROUPS. All of this analysis leads to the generalization that as children develop into pre-adolescents and on into teenagers they become more able to work productively in groups in classroom-directed learning activities. By high school, many youngsters can function in groups with a good deal of independence and can take themselves into some genuine experiences in learning. This is a process that will be possible to use throughout life, so becoming comfortable with it in school is a valuable health education experience.

AT LAST . . . THE PHYSICAL! Although commonly associated with the physical, the growing and developing concept belongs no more to the physical realm than to any other.

Growing and developing begins at conception with the merging of the nuclei of the sperm and the ovum and the alignment of chromosomes that precedes the first mitosis into two cells, then four, eight and . . . . There are a number of insults to the mother's physiology that can adversely affect the developing embryo . . . and then fetus . . . such as certain infections (measles) and drugs—both legal and illicit. We continue to make progress in identifying these hazards and preventing their occurrence or treating their aftermaths. The most obvious post-natal influence on developmental processes, however, is the size of the child at birth. Pregnancies average 280 days, but that exact time of conception often is impossible to ascertain. More importantly, pediatricians now know that the relative size of the baby at birth is the key factor. If it is below five and one-half pounds, it is considered premature, and the less it weighs the more growth and developmental problems it is likely to have throughout childhood—and life.

Physical growth is occurring as the child enters school and, again, not at the same rate for all youngsters, but with an assumed median regular steadiness, except in late childhood or early adolescence when a spurt is expected.

Development in the physical arena implies the increasing capacity to use, with effectiveness, the structures that have grown. Bones and muscles grow, and coordination in the use of these structures increases, with large muscle coordinations earlier than smaller muscle coordinations. Stamina also increases, so that longer and more sustained muscle activity is possible.

HANDEDNESS. Handedness is probably evident by the time the child comes to school. Since there are some obvious day-to-day advantages of being right-handed as the majority of Americans are, there are certain temptations to encourage a lefty to do more things with her/his right hand. Most medical authorities caution that the consequences can be worse than the condition. To work against the dominance pattern that is developing may leave the child uncertain and unskilled with either hand, and behind in many aspects of development. Now, obviously, some people must learn to use a non-dominant foot or hand, for some compelling reason, and since many do so without excessive trauma, there is no necessary tragedy with each relearning of handedness. Without a genuine reason for changing, however, the risk may not seem worth running.

CHEWING AND SMILING. Each youngster normally starts growing a set of baby teeth during the first year of life; these twenty small chewers develop and function during the first five or six years after birth, and then begin to loosen and fall out. The buds for the permanent teeth that now begin to appear formed before birth, but waited this dormant period before erupting. Since these are the teeth that the individual will have as a full-grown adult, they may look rather huge in a seven- or eight-year-old face. Growth and development in these teeth usually is rather normal, meaning that they present a fairly even and balanced smile and that they meet in a functional bite for chewing purposes. However, there are variations from the norm—children with missing teeth, too many teeth, crooked teeth, and teeth that do not meet and chew comfortably. The discomfort of these abnormalities may interfere with learning, or the self-consciousness and feelings of personal chagrin may work against full attention to learning, or the process of repair (braces, retainers, headbands, etc.) may detract, temporarily, from full learning. One unfortunately negative form of growing and developing is that of dental caries. The normal, accepted American diet and inadequate mouth care patterns encourage the development of tooth decay, which eventually becomes painful and distractive if not repaired. Because it is not now feasible for all children and youth to get the dental care they need (for the time being, at least), some must grow and develop adapting to whatever deficiencies are present.

OH, MY SKIN! The process of becoming an adolescent will be painfully evident in the facial skins of some young males and females. Unsightly blemishes, pimples, blackheads, and the most severe acne may make some youthful faces temporarily unattractive and, perhaps worse, cause amounts of anxiety and self-consciousness that definitely interfere with learning. Jeff and Nancy are slated to work together in a group tomorrow in their health class. Nancy, particularly, is looking forward to this chance to interact with Jeff. As she views herself in the morning mirror, she is horrified by the sight of a giant pimple right on her nose. If she doesn't go to school she obviously cannot learn from the experiences there; if she goes, her attention to the subject will almost certainly be limited by her worry over Jeff's reaction to this blazing defect. Most skins finally clear up as adulthood approaches, but some are irreparably scarred by this passage—as are some of the persons beneath the skins. Others, however, grow and develop a perspective on their mild disfigurement and lead full, happy lives despite the early damage. Some persons continue to have pimples. The attitude of "Nobody's perfect" can be a very healthy one.

BECOMING AN ATHLETE. Youth who develop above average coordination, stamina, and particular abilities may well become members of competitive athletic teams and grow and develop as athletes. This may be only a part of all-around development, or it may become a focus for time, interest, and attention that interferes with classroom learning. Many schools are so committed to all-around development for all students that they require a certain amount of success in the classroom as a prerequisite for athletic competition. This is supposed to stimulate a desire to achieve. If it does, fine; if it does not, the school is, in effect, saying, "If you do not succeed in Spanish and geometry, you may not succeed in anything." Retaining high standards in any realm of life inevitably produces some individual human casualties. Then must come the judgment: Is the standard worth the casualties? Whatever decision is made, it is rarely unanimous.

SEXUALITY. In contrast, as soon as the birth process is completed, it is nearly always possible to hold the baby up and get unanimous judgment that "It's a girl!" or "It's a boy!" The judgment is made, of course, on the absence of the small but prominent penile protuberance and its accompanying small scrotal sac and the presence, instead, of a set of labia between the legs. At birth and until puberty, these structures function more as urinary passages, but they presage the growing and developing of the individual into a physiologically, hormonally functioning sexual being. Actually, the conditioning for life as a male or female begins with the first perception and announcement ("It's a . . . ."). The baby is given a name (David or Dorothy), and certain colors and styles of garments seem more or less appropriate . . . then ribbons or no ribbons, lace or no lace . . . and then toys may begin to differentiate.

THE START OF SCHOOL. By the time youngsters start kindergarten or first grade, each has grown and developed as boy or girl. Oh, one could identify some girls who might be called tomboys and some boys who might be called sissies, which signify that in behavior the sexes definitely overlap. There have been times when length of hair has been a clear distinguishing factor of identifying males or females. There have been times when clothes worn to school constituted a differentiating factor; this is not one of those times . . . except if someone does wear a dress she is very probably a female. Males go to toilet rooms marked "Boys"; females go to ones marked "Girls." Girls' rooms have closed toilets. Boys' toilets have urinal space as well.

POTENTIAL DIFFERENCES DEVELOP INTO REAL. During the early elementary years, there are no general differences between girls and boys, except for their urination equipment . . . and their potentials. But by the fourth grade (oh, it could happen in the third), the T-shirts and tight dresses of a few girls are beginning to bulge a bit in the breast areas. By sixth grade, or about twelve years of age, most girls have symbolically passed puberty by beginning to menstruate, an indication that growing and developing has brought the reproductive system into functioning. Their hips widen. Hair grows under the arms and over the labia that covers the vagina between the legs (this is actually a form of fur, since it grows to a certain length and stops; no cutting, as for head hair, is necessary), Menstruation also brings on the cycle of female hormone production, responsible for the reproduction potential, for certain female characteristics, and, perhaps, for women's reduced susceptibility to heart and circulatory disease.

In boys, the pubertal changes come, on the average, a year and a half to two years later, but still far in advance of any need to use the reproductive system responsibly in our society. In boys, the penis enlarges in length and diameter and the scrotum and testicles inside enlarge. In no way is puberty marked as dramatically as with girls' menstruation. Puberty for boys is marked by the production and discharge of mature spermatozoa. Hair begins to grow under the arms and around the penis, and hair begins to grow on the face—the beginning, for most American males, of a lifetime of daily shaving. The muscular system, under the influence of the male hormones now being secreted, begins to harden and becomes capable of harder and longer work. The shoulders tend to widen, and the muscles tend to bulge more than those of females.

WE'RE ALL SOME OF EACH. In terms of sex hormone production, no one probably is, or has ever been, completely male or entirely female. We all are combinations, with even masculine males and feminine females being 80%-20%, or even 70%-30%. It also happens that there are some 60%-40%, who are identified as one sex or the other, but have many characteristics of the other—because they have a goodly supply of the "other" hormones. So, Benny is a male, but his muscles are rather soft (and he really does not desire to build them up), his breast tissue is more enlarged than that of most boys, his facial hair is sparse, and his voice just didn't deepen very much. Annie is a strapping, strong girl with wide shoulders and narrow hips. Her muscles are hard and well-developed. Her breasts are small and rarely interfere with her vigorous activities. She is hairier than most girls, with almost an embarrassing growth of hair on her upper lip. Her voice is low and powerful.

Now, the point to be made, without bothering to argue whether Benny and Annie are normal or not, is that post-pubertal humans who have strong male hormones are designed for physical work and vigorous exercise, with wide shoulders, narrow hips to make movement easier, bulky and/or supple muscles and minimal breast tissue to interfere with movement. There also may be more tendency to be aggressive, to tackle a hard job, and to fight for one's rights, but these certainly are learned behaviors. Thus, the influence of hormones probably cannot be measured accurately. Conversely, humans with strong female hormones are more inclined to have a soft, curvy musculature, large breast tissue, wider and fatter hips, and thus be less well designed for muscular effort. They also may be more passive, more compassionate, and less competitive, but these cannot be separated from learned behaviors. These probably are best called masculine and feminine extremes. Through most of our nation's history, these could be called norms for males and females, but with immediate concession that there were some exceptions.

NORMAL? Today, we are not sure what to call normal. There are strong forces to reduce the differences between normal growing and developing of boys and girls after puberty—to consider more behaviors as potentially normal that used to be considered deviant. Since we are not at all sure that labelling some person as different or abnormal did him/her or the society any good, we are justifiably trying out the opposite tack.

As sexual beings, however, boys and girls in late elementary, junior high and high school are growing and developing in their thinking about and imagining encounters with the opposite sex—some realistic . . . some fantasy. This imagining may sometimes be accompanied by masturbation as a fuller simulation of the sexual act. In encounters with members of the opposite sex, in talking with one's own sex-mate about sex and particularly representatives of the "opposite," and in experiencing some sexual situations, each individual is developing a pattern of behavior—as sexually aggressive, sexually shy, sexually promiscuous, sexually selective or sexually receptive. Such patterns always can be changed, but to the extent that if any one is repeatedly reinforced, it tends to produce predictable behavior, unless real effort is made to change.

REPRODUCTION POTENTIAL. If we had universally effective contraception for all unmarried post-pubertal girls, the sexual system (the penis and clitoris-vagina) and the reproductive system (testes-spermatozoa and uterus-Fallopian tubes-ovaries-ovum) would be functionally independent. The fact is that at puberty both boys and girls grow and develop instantly into humans capable of the physiological process of reproduction. However, emotional, mental, and social growth into a possibly effective parent is always a much longer process. Typically, the sexual system is going to be exercised before it is desirable for the reproductive system to function (in marriage as well as before).

SEX DISTRACTS. So, what does this add up to? Growing and developing as a sexual being often is a distractor from learning. In a relatively free choice, competitive system of dating, courtship and marriage such as ours, where dating and pairing off begin about midway through the school experience, the school setting becomes a natural arena for this activity. It is often much more compelling of attention than classroom activities. There is still no agreement among school people or among health personnel that education about this developing sexuality is a proper part of health education. Much opposition seems to center on the issue of whether the health teacher can do it well enough. Some protest that this should be a private educational experience between parent and child . . . perhaps with the help of clergy. Others contend that medical training is an essential prerequisite, while others, going not so far, still argue that a sex educator should be especially educated and trained . . . beyond that of the typical health teacher. No resolution of this controversy seems to be in sight.

IN SUMMARY, then, educators must accept the fact that developing sexuality, dating, sexual fantasizing, feelings of guilt and shame over sexual acts, planning for more sexual activity, actual premarital pregnancy, and actual or suspected venereal disease are going to be generally negative influences on achievement in school. This is an educational realm all its own, and most young people will consider it more important, at least at times, than causes of accidents, the Four Food Groups, and quacks and nostrums you should avoid . . . .

Growing and developing is going on when the child enters school, and the school experience encompasses the important development from child to adolescent to young adult. The school has to assume some general, steady progress in most growing and developing, and then do what it can to help those who depart from the expected norm. Growing and developing can proceed in a number of ways, but when a student develops a pattern and reinforces it, it becomes difficult to change. The opportunities for change can come in interacting and decision-making. "How . . . ?" you surely do ask.

INTERACTING is actively responding in some dimension or combination of dimensions to things happening around one. In the intellectual realm, it refers to a person experiencing both abstract and concrete facts, ideas, and concepts and really dealing with these in some eventually apparent way. Let's reintroduce the example involving beer expressed earlier in the chapter. Some young children interact first with the abstraction or the idea of beer from commercials, billboards, etc. The first interaction of other tots is more with the beverage itself—with beer cans, bottles, glasses emptied by parents or other adults, and even with an occasional sip from the nearly empty can or glass. Later comes interacting with the concept of beer drinking, with moderation and excess, with happy and sad results from drinking. Then may come the interacting in becoming or not becoming a beer drinker—with beer, with drinking friends, with non-drinking folk, with the law, with conscience and self-concept. . . . These situations for interacting probably continue throughout life, influencing and being influenced by the growing and developing process in relation to beer.

Memorizing is another interesting intellectual interaction. We read and hear many combinations of words each day, and, if we interact with them, we may remember certain generalizations, particular phrases or numbers, but the exact words quickly fade away. Memorizing thus requires a particular kind of sustained interacting so that the result is the capacity to repeat something word-for-word, perhaps even in a particular predictable style. My second son was recently awarded the role of Henry Higgins in his school's musical, "My Fair Lady." The lines and speeches he must memorize are certainly many, coupled with the task of uttering them with the proper British accent . . . and, eventually, saying them in interacting with Liza, Pickering and other characters in the play.

Reasoning and developing concepts are other examples of mental interacting. These are somewhat difficult processes, so no one applies his/her reason to every situational experience. And from where does whatever capacity the individual has come? From the continuing interaction of the hereditary potential of the young person with the total environment and with certain specific portions thereof, that's where. Studies in American education generally suggest that Max, who grows up in a home where newspapers, magazines, and books are evident, where ideas and curiosity in knowing are valued, and where education is, in many direct and indirect ways, lauded, will have a greater developed capacity to learn than Teddy. Teddy's home is barren of written materials, conversations are functional or perjorative, and his parents and other home-mates look upon and describe school education as a "drag." However, all kids coming out of Max-type homes are not of the same ability or achievement—nor are those from the Teddy-type nest. To exhibit the democratic principle, a sister of Teddy may be brighter and achieve more in school than one of Max's siblings. However, the generalization stands: a favorable environment helps develop all levels of innate ability . . . and the more ability, the more it can be developed. Conversely, a barren or unfavorable environment is very tough to overcome, even for the individual with hereditary ability.

CAN'T INTERACT WITH EVERYTHING. In any environment, an individual only interacts with some of the stimuli available. In the classroom, Mandy interacts some of the time with the teacher, with other students, with books, bulletin boards, sounds, smells and with other stimuli. Some of these encourage learning according to the curriculum, some detract from learning, and some encourage other kinds of non-curricular learning. Mandy also interacts with symbols and suggestions of success, failure and with no recognition or no indication of success or failure. Each tends to produce emotions, particularly if Mandy has learned to compete; even if she is not very competitive, the interacting with other students who do compete will probably produce some emotions. And those emotions begin to interact with other emotions . . . and with the emotions of others. . . .

EMOTIONAL ENCOUNTERS. School, then, is a series of interactions nearly always involving some combination of emotions and reasons. No one can ever be sure what the balance is for Mandy, for Matt, or for any supposed learner, but behavior may be a helpful key. If Mandy is using three reference books and writing her section of a group report, it appears that the balance is toward reason. If Matt is angrily carving up his plastic desk top, it appears that emotion is on top. If Elizabeth sits passively and watches a film . . . who knows? However, in another situation Mandy may appear to be paying attention, but actually is thinking about the puppies born to her bitch the night before. Matt may appear to be sullen and disinterested, but is actually paying as much attention as he can.

A GAME TO PLAY. Another complication in evaluating behavior directly as representative of feeling is what I shall call "The Game of Adult and Child." This is not to be equated with the transactional analysis framework for therapy. Also, it is not to be confused with gaming, an acceptable educational approach to get learners to apply information and make decisions. In this game, the adult appears to expect more accomplishments and less mischief than she/he knows is possible or likely, while the youngsters appear to "fool around" more than they should. Adults thus set standards and exert discipline a bit beyond what they expect, and youngsters try to take more liberties than they usually want. If the game goes well, a balance of behavior results that is reasonably satisfying to all. But because it is partly or perhaps nearly wholly an unconscious game, individuals may get it badly out of whack.

INTERACTING WITH SELF . . . AND OTHERS. As argued earlier, the school and the home generally hope that self-discipline will grow and develop in the learner during the school years. Outside forces can exert discipline and can encourage self-discipline, but the latter really develops out of the individual interacting with her/himself, the essence of which is achieving the goal or overcoming short term distractions in favor of some more important objective. At this moment, I am struggling to write this instead of entering into a fascinating conversation very close to me. It appears at this moment that self-discipline is winning!

In the bigger picture, each Dick and Jane is continually interacting with self—in seeing and perceiving, in judging, in comparing . . . in balancing one desire with others. However, one can become a really whole and functioning person only by interacting also with other fellow humans. During the child's early years of necessary dependence, much of the interaction is rather structured. Cindy falls down, skins her knee, cries, runs into the house, and Mother comforts her, washes the knee, and puts on a Band-Aid. As attempts at independence begin, the interactions become less structured and predictable and yet more real. As the individual reaches the maturity of interdependence, she/he is then in the longest life stage of complete interacting—independent interacting, interacting with people semi-structured, and interacting with people in very structured ways.

In a classroom setting, a group project has the potential for the most interacting. If a heterogeneous group of eighth graders, for instance, selects their own topic, decides how they will gather information and how they will present it, divides responsibilities (utilizing each in her/his best ways), and actually presents the results in some creative way, there has been a whale of a lot of personal interacting, intra-group interacting with learning processes, and with the subject matter. Such an educational experience has the greatest potential for memorable success . . . and also the greatest possibility of being a disaster.

Interacting within peer groups, not selected within a classroom and not necessarily task-oriented, constitutes much of the interacting life of many children and youth. Some youngsters appear quite consistent; in any group they are in they are likely to feel and behave in consistent fashion. Others are more adaptable, emphasizing different facets of personality with different groups. Depending on your value context (and perhaps on your own life-style), you think more highly of the consistent person or the adaptable person. There undoubtedly is some merit in each.

PHYSICAL INTERACTING. The first interacting of consequence to any individual is that between an ovum and a particular spermatozoon (out of hundreds of millions "in the neighborhood"), which form a zygote, which interacts with the Fallopian tube, the chemical environment and then the uterus to form a viable pregnancy. After nine months or so, a complex interacting results in the birth of the child. After birth, appropriate interacting results in growth and development, physical interactions such as moving, pushing, throwing and kicking. Most youngsters begin to interact consistently in using one hand and foot (and eye), usually the right, more than the other.

Teeth develop, and the child interacts by using them . . . and as they are used, they tend to become stronger. A smile likely makes an interaction more pleasant. Particular interacting with sugars in the mouth results in cavities. The skin of some adolescents interacts with some chemicals, some foods, or some kinds of care . . . and breaks out in blemishes, blotches, or whatever. Interacting with others, particularly the smooth-faced, that becomes more risky.

ATHLETIC ENCOUNTERS. Some adolescents become athletes. They perform in commendable fashion in sports and, consequently, begin to interact with others as athletes. They not only learn the movements and successful styles for a particular sport, but they learn terminology, records, plays, and strategies. They become emotionally related to a game or sport, and they may associate, socially, with others of like commitment. These can be powerful interactions. As part of my first teaching job, I helped, on two occasions, coach an all-star football team from the Honolulu Interscholastic League. One team was made up of the best players from four teams, and the other composed of the best players from the other four teams. One year, for instance, there were middle and upper class Caucasians from a private prep school, Hawaiian kids from the school for part-Hawaiians, middle and lower class Japanese from one public school, and low income Filipinos, Portuguese, and racial mixtures from another public school. They assembled as just young people. They were very ill at ease and uncomfortable, but as they put on equipment they began to interact more positively. As they practiced together and impressed each other with prowess, interactions became easier. When they all put on identical All-Star uniforms and saw themselves in opposition to others in different uniforms, the interacting became one of genuine camaraderie, spectacularly different from that of less than two weeks before. Athletic competition is more than just organized physical exercise. It is experience that athletes have, and non-athletes do not have. It is a way of thinking and acting. It is a kind of role that can carry over into social and personal life apart from the actual competition. It can be helpful; it can be harmful; as you might expect, it can be some of each.

BOY-GIRL INTERACTIONS. As noted earlier, some decisions are made as to whether a baby is a girl or a boy, and interacting begins with that as a premise. Children are directly and subtly taught "how girls are" and "how boys are" and what appropriate interactions are. There are exceptions to the norm, but they are generally regarded as exceptions rather than another form of the norm. Byron knits instead of playing kickball; parents of other boys like and accept Byron, but most of them would want their own boys to play kickball rather than knit. Janice is on the rifle team; parents of other girls may like and accept Janice, but most of them would prefer that their own girls be song or cheer leaders, in dramatics, in swimming . . . something more feminine than being on the rifle team. So boys and girls learn early, before any significant differences in hormones appear, that there are expected differences between males and females. One study, in the last decade, reported that elementary teachers (mostly females) tended to touch and caress in friendly fashion girls significantly more than boys. This could be an important factor in learning differences between the sexes.

At puberty, however, the differential production of male and female sex hormones begins, and the interactions between female and male take on a whole new quality. Girls begin to menstruate, a reaction of the uterine wall to an ovum produced that is not fertilized and implanted. But this physical happening can produce a wider range of interactions. Hear this after-school report from my son Ricky when he was in the fifth grade:

> Today the girls got to see a movie, but the boys didn't . . . we wanted to know what it was about . . . I asked Terry afterwards, but she said she couldn't tell me . . . I saw her showing something written in her notebook to another girl, so I chased her and threw her down and tried to see what it was, but she fought hard and wouldn't let me see . . . the teacher made me let her up.

As parents we responded:

> The film was about menstruation . . . showing girls why they are or will soon be beginning to bleed from the vagina for a few days each month.

He responded:

> How do you spell and say that word?

We showed and told him. The next afternoon he said:

> I showed the word to Terry and asked her if that was the one. She said it was . . . I don't see why girls get to see that movie and we don't . . . .

Perhaps this symbolizes the fat fact that the physiological changes that come with puberty are responsible, in this culture, for a lot of interactions—some expected, but some distorted, frenzied, aggressive, competitive. . . .

Boy-girl interactions involve a panoply of sensations—seeing, hearing, smelling . . . later touching and testing . . . all related and stirred around by imagination and the capacity to fantasize. While the passage of the female into puberty (menstruation) is a more physically obvious occurrence than comparable passage for the male, the situation is reversed when it comes to outward manifestation of stimulation by the opposite sex. For an adolescent boy, a picture of an attractive girl, the sight and smell of a girl, the mind-picture of a girl, and particularly close body contact with a girl can bring on an erection of the penis and heightened sexual feelings, since these are more centralized in the genitals of the male than of the female. The adolescent girl, however attracted, has no such physical interactive response to indicate to anyone her attraction.

SEXUAL INTERACTIONS INTERFERE WITH STUDY. There are many, many examples of interacting that could be described or alluded to, but the central criterion for this chapter of this book should be those that affect learning in the classroom. Coeducational secondary schools are educational institutions but they also are dating and courtship institutions, where required attendance offers many opportunities for making acquaintances that will be developed more fully outside of school. Sometimes these boy-girl interactions develop around some academic task (studying for a test or doing a project together) or around some other school-related activity (putting out the yearbook, putting on a musical production) where the accomplishment of the task may actually be abetted. The other obvious result to be noted is that personal interactions between opposite sexes are often at the expense of school learning. An individual can only interact with—give attention to—a limited number of stimuli at one time. Thinking about whether Tony really likes you more than he does Cleo may be more absorbing than learning the seven danger signals of cancer or why there are so many interpretations of a good diet regimen. If Sandy has to interact with her parents, siblings, chores at home, her three boyfriends, a part-time job, responsibilities in a club, participation on an athletic team and with five different, often competing, school subjects, it is easy to see why each teacher does not receive her full and best interaction.

GOAL-LEARNING. One last important observation, however. The task of the school—and of health education—is to encourage each learner to interact with some new information, ideas and concepts, and some new ways of learning so that future life interacting will be from a wider base, and one's decisions can be the results of a broader range of considerations.

And, thus, the third key concept is introduced: decision-making. All forms of life grow and develop, and all forms interact, but only the human being has decision-making as an aspect of total functioning. Many lower life forms make choices and show evidences of intelligence. People's capacity to decide to do one thing rather than another based on some knowledge of the past, an assessment of the present, and some predictions of the future, combined with a valuing process, provides them with a not entirely unique, but certainly a distinctive, dimension of health. It is our cultural belief in this decision-making capacity that undergirds our strong commitment to education and, specifically, health education.*

If people, all throughout life, make decisions that are based on what they know and how they feel, then the more they know and the more conscious they are of why they have certain feelings, the more decisions are apt to produce desirable results. Another premise behind health education is that individuals are not so unique and self-contained that they cannot learn from the experiences of others—and particularly from those experiences that are systematically evaluated and analyzed and called science. So, for example, we have some faith in the premise that some young non-smokers will not become smokers because carefully gathered and analyzed data suggest that those who smoke develop lung cancer, emphysema, and heart disease more frequently than non-smokers. In other words, those young learners who accept the facts of the hazards of smoking feel that this is undesirable and that the future

---

* It may be important to note that the conviction that one has, in fact, made a decision is a philosophical, non-provable assumption. There are other old and new traditions, from Hinduism to B. F. Skinner, that have much less commitment to the reality of apparent choice-making. For the final, unanswerable question to a statement such as "I decided to buckle my seat belt today" is "How do you know you could have done any other—on this day at this time? If you did it, then you may have been able to do no other." These competing traditions obviously believe in forces more powerful than the individuals that control what they do, completely or in part. Proof or non-proof is based on agreement as to what is valid proof, and this finally is based on assumption and belief.

hazards are more important than present desirable smoking behavior. All learners do not meet all these qualifications, but some undoubtedly do. And health educators are happiest with those who do.

RELATIONSHIPS TO OTHER KEYS. How does decision-making fit in with the other concepts of growing and developing and interacting? Oversimplified, the ways that an individual has grown and developed to a particular time and place influence greatly how she/he makes a decision then and there. In turn, the decision made and carried out serves to reinforce or to counter a pattern of growing and developing. Then, too, decision-making comes out of interacting in situations.

Mike gets up late and must eat hurriedly if he is to get to school on time. There are three boxes of cereal on the shelf and he fairly arbitrarily picks the middle one; the cereal is not one he dislikes so he pours a bowl of it. He really has not made a decision; he has chosen one over two others, but there were no significant criteria . . . he did not really think about it much. In a moment, however, he finds there are containers of both whole milk and non-fat milk in the refrigerator. He normally would just pour from the whole milk container without much thought, but yesterday there was a debate in his health class. He had been on the team defending the practices of eating the foods you really like, whether they're best for you or not. One of the subject issues had been milk, and though he had defended the use of whole milk if you liked it, he had listened to the arguments for milk with less saturated fat, particularly for postpubescent males. All of this commands his attention at this moment standing in the open refrigerator door, and he decides to try the non-fat milk. On the cereal, it seems to taste little different from the whole milk, so this decision, based in some part upon a health education experience, may herald a small change in a growing and developing pattern. Perhaps in a year he would be interactively selecting the non-fat milk every time; or perhaps he still would be making decisions, sometimes one, sometimes the other.

In the example given, Mike seemed to have learned something he had not decided to learn. Decision-making is still much involved with what we do learn. Another day in Mike's health class was devoted to the question, "What will the drug scene be like five years from now?" Mike had some ideas, but he decided that he wasn't satisfied with these alone and did some fairly intensive reading of published predictions, and interviewed two people in his town who are involved with the current drug scene. In this way, he learned some things because he decided that he needed to.

DECIDING HOW TO USE LEARNING. Once knowledge is gained, then decisions about use arise. Do I just think about it? Do I tell others? Do I try to get others to really understand it? Do I translate it into behavior? Do I let this change my life-style? And any decision begs a bunch of other potentials. You probably suspected that I would try to get one more use out of that beer-drinking example, didn't you? Okay, let's say Denise has grown and developed at age 15, interacting occasionally with the "out-there" phenomenon of beer drinking—as something some others do. Now she is at an afternoon-evening picnic in an old stone quarry with an older boy she never has dated before. He pops a can of beer and hands it to her, and the decision is upon her. "No, thanks" symbolizes the decision to continue her abstinence. "Thanks" symbolizes the decision at least not to appear to be a total abstainer. But this leads on to other decisions . . . to drink some or not? . . . how fast and in what quantities? . . . to pretend that this is not the first time? . . . to have another? . . . if so, how soon? . . . to take part in any drinking games? . . . and so on.

BY HEART? Back to the academic realm for a comment on memorizing. Not much is memorized without some conscious decision to do so, because memorization typically requires a conscious directing of attention. To truly memorize anything of any length or substance requires continuously deciding that the result will be worth the effort . . . as worthwhile as other possible uses of time. The larger quality (of which memory is a part) of self-discipline is developed only as the result of many conscious decisions about directing attention.

The emotional realm is a fascinating one with reference to decision-making. The most obvious relation is that emotions influence certain decisions.

- Coach Pryor is angry and frustrated with his team's performance so he decides to have them practice for four hours on Saturday.
- Jerry is envious of Benny's new bike and decides he is going to work out some way to get one like it for his own.
- Penny feels so good today that she decides to write happy notes to her three old unmarried aunts who enjoy hearing from her.
- Alex is so in love with Kath that he decides to ask her to marry him.
- . . . and so on.

The other important thing to say is that many people make many decisions about controlling emotions that they may or may not be able to carry through. Actually most of us cannot consciously control emotions—"I will not hate. . . ." "I will not be jealous of. . . ." "I will love. . . ." We can decide, however, not to behave as a negative emotion would push us or to try to behave in a loving, forgiving fashion. This leads into the mental health issue as to whether it is better to express the emotions one feels or to suppress emotions and act only reasonably and calmly . . . or how any individual balances these options.

DEPENDENCE. The period of dependence in the life of a child is pretty generally a period when other people make decisions for her/him or where the decisions allowed are very simple and repetitive. Independence, then, is defined very much in terms of making one's own decisions and living with the consequences of them. That awkward period that many late elementary and secondary school youngsters find themselves in is one of making independent decisions but not being required to live with the consequences. But there is no way that parents can prevent their children from wanting to make independent decisions before they really are able. Decision-making needs to be practiced; it rarely springs forth fully developed in a young human.

Interdependence, the condition of maturity previously described, involves the combination of making independent decisions and living with the decisions made by someone else for you. The temptation to feel that "I am happiest with the decisions I make" must be adulterated with the feeling "Well, I wouldn't have decided to do that . . . but, it may turn out all right after all."

Well, what do you know . . . this has led us into decision-making about social relationships—about whom to relate to, whom to avoid, how, and why. These are probably the toughest decisions to make because people, particularly in groups, typically cannot be predicted with accuracy. For instance, groups are likely to be made up of some people who make personal decisions with great consistency and others who are inconsistent, to a greater or lesser degree. Arnold has moved to a new city with his family and is attending his first party. He is trying to determine, while socializing, whether this is one group or some gathering of somewhat compatible sub-groups. Before he can be at all sure, one of the girls whom he had pegged as "pretty square" asks him to join a small group smoking some "grass." He isn't sure whether this is normative for the whole group, whether they're going to pressure him to smoke, or whether they're testing him out and would respect a decision to decline. Arnold wishes, painfully, that he knew some of these things, but circumstances require him to make some decision now, with what he has surmised to this point. He may or may not ever find out how intuitive he was about what to do and how.

GROUP PRESSURE!? WHO NEEDS WHOM? A general rule about individuals and groups is this: if a group wants an individual to join them (because he/she is an athlete, has a sense of humor, is a good student . . . is attractive, is personable . . .) that individual can make and execute decisions about behavior according to personal standards, going with or against the group; the valuable person can set her/his own standards and may influence others in the group. On the other hand, if another individual needs the group more than it needs her/him, then she/he is under more pressure to behave in established ways. The peripheral person feels more need to decide in ways acceptable to group leaders. And within groups, there probably will always be some of each.

One of the most important situational decisions (and decision-making patterns) is that of how to use one's time. There obviously are many ways you and I can use each block of time. I could be doing at least seven things other than writing this page, and you probably have comparable alternatives to reading these well-chosen words. Actually, this use of time is a good example of an ever-changing combination of decision-making and interacting. I shall never forget the winter morning I decided, with great finality, to write a letter that was long overdue. I was progressing nicely on my self-appointed task when I noticed that the house was on fire, so I abandoned my original plan and spent considerable time making and carrying out decisions to save the old farmhouse. The letter was finished another day.

SEX-RELATED DECISIONS. Decision-making on the basis of sex still has some reality, but it certainly has become less clearcut over the past decade. Choices of casual and recreational clothing are affected less and less by the sex of the chooser, except, as noted, that males rarely wear skirts or dresses. A boy may decide to hitchhike across the state; a girl may decide to go with him. And her parents may decide not to try to prevent her from going. For the past two years, my son Mike has participated in a survival-type camp called "Underway," with obstacle courses, repelling off rock cliffs, hikes through dense forests, canoeing down some rapids, etc. One of the leaders told me that they have groups of girls in some of the camp periods, and that they accomplish the whole program as well as, and sometimes better than, groups of boys. In choosing careers the notion that some are just for men, others just for women is eroding fast. Police departments increasingly have some arresting officers who are female . . . at least matched in the culture by some male nurses and kindergarten teachers. The fascinating (though not necessarily important) question in this context is, Are we really deciding to make these changes toward equality, or are a few pushing hard for change and the rest just interacting?

Relations between post-pubertal females and males certainly involve a lot of interacting, but also some decisions. A boy may have to decide what girl to ask to the Saturday picnic; then, how to ask her; then, what to do when she turns him down. . . . A girl may have to decide how to get the boy she likes to ask her to the picnic; then, how to stall another boy until she knows whether her choice is going to ask her; then, how direct she should be in seeing that she goes with whom she wants. . . . Some decision-making situations are not new:

Should I kiss a boy on a first date?
but the answer may be
Only if he's with you!

PHYSICAL DECISIONS. The context, of course, is that adolescent boys and girls have come out of childhood where close body contact with the opposite sex had no erotic communication. Most are on their way to adulthood and to at least one relationship of complete sexual intimacy. So, though there are many potential decisions, the giant one is still, probably, Should I have sexual intercourse?—with the possible corollary, With or without some means of preventing pregnancy? How such decisions are made and carried out does still affect the educational achievements of some young people.

IN SUMMARY. Young learners, the clientele for school health education, are growing and developing, in some common ways, in some ways like others, and in some ways quite uniquely. This is affected by ways each individual interacts and by decisions made. The mental dimension of well-being obviously is an important affector of learning, but so are the educational, the social, and the physical. In one sense, we can see that childhood and youth is a time for maximum learning about healthful living, and yet in another sense, some aspects of living interfere with maximum learning.

Characteristics of learners vary according to how they grow and develop mentally, emotionally, socially, and physically.

Some growing and developing is positive and productive, and some makes it difficult or impossible for a youngster to function well as a learner.

Learning is a matter of interacting with processes and subject content; other interactions—emotional, social, and physical—sometimes assist, and sometimes detract.

Interacting between males and females in the school setting is natural and inevitable, but may interfere with learning.

The ultimate concept related to learning is decision-making, the learner's capacity to exert will to learn, in competition with other calls for the use of time and attention.

Chapter V

Health Education: Science and Non-Science

Some of the content of this chapter typically is not said in books of this type. It is meant to inform, not to inflame. It is intended as a widener of perspective on both our present and our past.

Many of the original colonists of this nation had fled religious persecution in Britain or Europe, but were in no more harmonious agreement with neighbors here than they had been there. So the Constitution proclaimed that there should be no establishment of an official religion. It was not so much that Americans were non-religious, but that they represented a diversity of religious and sectarian beliefs and practices, and this diversity has been seen as strength.

SUPERNATURAL FORCES. Though our money is still imprinted with the affirmation "In God We Trust," and courtroom witnesses and elected government officials take oaths that ask for God's help in what they are about to do, the official governmental structure and function of our society is not religious.

A culture in which governmental functioning reflects an official religion is a theocracy. Our founding fathers, recognizing the right of individuals to believe as they wish, the necessity for public officials to make decisions for all the people, and the excesses of past theocracies, chose to separate church and state . . . "rendering unto Caesar that which is Caesar's and to God that which is God's."

To make the contrast clearer, hear some expressions of individual belief that cannot be a basis for deliberations of State.

"All illness, disability, and premature death result from sin . . . not measuring up to God's expectations."

"Everything that happens is God's will . . . what He does not directly cause He allows . . . this includes illness, disability, and premature death."

"Illness, disability, and premature death often result from karma or moral retribution . . . things happen to people because they have to happen . . . a result of sin in some former life on earth."

"God is the only healer . . . pray to God, and if it is His will He will answer the prayer and bring about healing."

And further, public education being by and for all citizens cannot reflect such beliefs as the following:

"All Knowledge, all wisdom is in God . . . study His word, pray, and meditate, and He will teach you all you need to know."

"Studying the Scriptures is the means to all learning of any importance."

"The important things are learned through revelation . . . they are revealed to those who wait upon the Lord."

"The most important focus for learning is the influence of God in human history."

MEDICINE AS SCIENCE. Modern medicine, now considered to be both art and science, has largely supplanted folk medicine in American culture. Its fundamental premises are: (1) there are natural (in contrast to supernatural) causes for all departures from health; (2) modes of diagnosis and treatment to be used are those that have been tested scientifically and proven best; and (3) the physicians' art and skill should be supplemented by technology, providing medicines and equipment to aid the healing process. Science is based on the assumptions that (1) nature has a somewhat predictable order; (2) this is discoverable and quantifiable; and (3) this knowing how and why something is as it is enables one to change or modify it. The rock base of science is the experiment. Example: In order to determine whether a particular fertilizer affects the growth of tomatoes, Dr. John Roe selects two fields, identical in soil composition, sunlight, wind, rainfall . . . in everything that could also affect the tomato growing. The tomatoes planted must be of the same seed source, with seeds randomly selected for each plot. One field is treated with the fertilizer, and the other one, the control, is not. Tomatoes are planted and care of the two plots must be exactly the same, except for the application of fertilizer to one plot. Dr. Roe then sets some criteria for measuring differences in tomatoes. The easiest and most quantifiable would be numbers of tomatoes and size in diameter and weight. Other, more subjective criteria might be susceptibility to insect damage, firmness, texture, and, more importantly from the standpoint of the tomato's use, taste. He then observes carefully and systematically keeps his data in an orderly form. Being a good scientist, he proposes the null hypothesis—that there will be no difference between the tomatoes from the two plots. He already has set an end to the experiment . . . or at some point he declares it finished and totals up the measurements. If he finds at the end of the experiment that the differences between the tomatoes could not have occurred by chance more than five times in any hundred trials. he concludes, announces, and publishes that the fertilizer does in fact cause the production of more, bigger, and heavier tomatoes. Following successful replication of the experiment by others, the conclusion can be drawn and the world informed, via science, that fertilizer helps tomatoes.

Actually, all we really know is that under certain conditions there was a particular result, and, if these conditions were to be replicated exactly 100 different times, the result would be like the original 95 times. We then must decide, by judgment rather than scientific measurement, whether another situation is enough like the experiment to expect comparable results.

WHY THE TOMATOES? This example was chosen purposefully. To illustrate a classic scientific experiment, it would have been better to choose a test tube experiment in a laboratory. In a tomato plot, one cannot control all variables as well as in the lab, and the criteria for success are partly subjective. But the tomato plot can be controlled with greater precision than can the patients at a clinic or the students in a classroom. Our culture does not approve of subjecting human patients to the controls necessary for rigid scientific experimentation. This greatly limits the conclusions of people-research and their generalizability.

THE COMPROMISE is a lot of evidence from clinical research. The medical researcher hypothesizes that a particular form of treatment would be effective against a particular malady or set of symptoms. For some period of time, she/he treats all such symptoms with this remedy and tries to keep records to show the results. The treatment is not being compared against no treatment; its evaluation is more. Do patients utilizing it lose their symptoms and get well? Again, this can be controlled best in a hospital or other custodial setting. Physicians practicing out of an office or clinic rarely have chances to follow up on patients unless they return . . . and there is no way to control the myriad other factors that make one person's illness different from another's illness.

MOTHER NATURE MAY NOT KNOW BEST. Technology makes scientific findings useful. Scientists discover how to develop an insulin that can bring relative normality back to the lives of diabetics; technology makes it possible for diabetics in Omaha, Tacoma, and Vero Beach to have insulin to take daily. The science of optics develops lenses that correct many forms of aberrant vision; technology means that most people who need them can get a pair of comfortable, useful glasses. The emphasis in science and technology is on helping nature when nature seems to be favoring human well-being and on combatting nature when it seems to be eroding human well-being. The emphasis in science is not on acceptance of nature "as is" nor on acceptance of nature's right to favor other forms of life over human beings at certain times.

For medicine, then, we, as a culture, favor a naturalistic-scientific outlook. However, nature is something to manipulate if it is not favorable to people, and science is a good way of knowing as long as it does not involve clashing with other values.

IN EDUCATION, the agricultural model for research (two plots of tomatoes with fertilizer in one) has been a dominant one in determining the efficacy of various approaches to learning. If the evaluative criteria are simple, like learning to add numbers or recognize words (or produce heavier tomatoes), scientific experiments can show superior and inferior approaches. However, if the question is, Are young learners better people after this learning experience? (comparable to, Are the fertilized tomatoes better all-around tomatoes?), then scientific investigation has not been of much help in improving the teaching-learning process. To be truly scientific in relation to education is usually quite difficult because the variables represented by a class of 35 individuals plus one or more teachers involved in something that occupies a small portion of their total daily time are simply unknown and uncontrollable.

The School Health Education Study was applauded by Dr. Ole Sand,[1] Director of the National Education Association's Center for the Study of Instruction in the middle 1960's as "an excellent example of rational planning in curriculum. . . ." He noted that the Study had carried out an essential first step—a nationwide status study to determine how students were achieving and what administrators were believing about health instruction programs. This status study, an enormous job, showed that students did not know all of the things they should have and were more knowledgeable in some areas than in others, that students did not have all the right attitudes, and that students do not behave in ways deemed healthful all the time. It also indicated that there were not many really going health education programs. These undoubtedly were good things to find out, but they did not lead, necessarily, to the development of a conceptual approach to curriculum design. As a matter of fact, this conceptual approach was taken primarily because curriculum projects in other fields such as mathematics, biology, chemistry . . . were concept-centered, but none of them had begun with a status study. The main point, I suppose, is that a scientific study never tells you what to do; it tells you what is . . . or what was, under certain given circumstances . . . that generates some hypothesis based on other values for dealing with the finding.

I CAN'T CONTROL THE VARIABLES! Let me repeat the major difficulty in being scientific in real life: many of the variables cannot be identified, controlled, or their effects be accurately accounted for in interpreting results. This seriously limits their generalizability and practical usefulness. Medicine deals with the whole person, but the initial focus

---

[1] School Health Education Study Writing Group, *Health Education.* pg. 10.

is often on some aspect of the physical, the easiest dimension about which to be scientific. Education also is concerned with the total being, but the main thrust is often on the mental-rational-intellectual dimension that, in itself, is also fairly easy to deal with scientifically. It is the emotional, social, aesthetic, and spiritual dimensions that don't seem to meet the scientific dictum. Anything that exists, exists in quantity; anything that exists in quantity can be measured.

SOME NON-SCIENCE. People—and that's what patients and learners are—are only partly scientific. Most people have some amount of a pragmatic spirit—trying something to see if it works and valuing that which works—which is the true spirit of technology. But the folk who make up even an educated nation generate other explanations also. Hear some of them:

- Why did it happen to her? Just kinda fate, I think. Something like this was bound to happen to her . . . for some reason.
- Jim survived and is walking around healthy today because he's one of the luckiest guys I know. Good luck just smiles on him!
- Why did it happen? Just circumstances . . . it wasn't anybody's fault, really. Just circumstances . . . crazy circumstances.
- Why was she the one that it happened to? Just chance. With all the people exposed it was bound to affect some. By chance, it was Gladys.

All of these unscientific views eschew the need for a clear delineated cause and blame. They credit something rather supernatural, orderly or whimsical, predictable or completely not. The explanations are easier, and most of us, however well-educated, have some tendencies to respond in some or all of these ways. Probably because however completely and thoroughly a mishap may be analyzed and explained as to causes, it seems as though the causative factors do not always a mishap make. For example, after a party where there has been much consumption of alcoholic drinks, seven cars leave, all the drivers in some state of intoxication. One car has an accident and six do not. Sure, the circumstances were different for each, but investigation probably would not show great differences between the experience that resulted in the accident and those that made it. The alcohol will be considered a major causative factor (which it may have been . . . it certainly has the potential), but it was also present in the non-accidents. Why the difference? The temptation may be strong to call on fate, luck (good or bad), circumstances, and/or chance. Perhaps consideration should also be given to the many possible variables that can contribute to accidents.

SOME EXAMPLES. Rare is the person who lives entirely and consistently according to scientific findings because non-scientific practices and styles of life are fairly widespread. They are spread from person to person because of friendship, trust in siblings, peers, and even adults.

There are recommended ways to select a physician when one moves to a new community. One should contact the county medical society and get names, and one should investigate medical training and subsequent experience and decide on some objective basis. But how much more frequent is the conversation with a new friend, that included, ". . . we've gone to Dr. Crouse for several years and we really like him . . . but don't go to Mulligan!" If the person seems compatible in other ways, the advice may be translated to a potentially very important behavior.

It is interesting and ironic that as science supplants religion as the ultimate trusted way of knowing in this culture, it develops in some strangely similar ways. Pure science should be the antithesis of dogmatism. In pure science, nothing should be taken without question; even scientific findings must be verified; new findings may require a whole reassembling of generalizations. Truth is only what has been shown to be consistently proved and verified. But the dogma of science is in its method. It is most intolerant of approaches to truth other than the scientific method. The superiority of a method rather naturally leads to superiority of truth obtained by that method. Perhaps the general public has demanded it, or perhaps the temptation upon scientists was, and is, too great to resist . . . for whatever combination of reasons, science has become our secular authority.

The anthropologist Francis L. K. Hsu[2] summed up a report entitled "A Cholera Epidemic in a Chinese Town" with the observation that the Chinese in the village had a magic-religious way of coping with diseases, and though they did some medically sound things, they did them for their own reasons. ". . . to achieve popular acceptance, magic has to be dressed like science in America, while science has to be cloaked as magic in Hsi-ch'eng." In American culture, we are more apt to believe and to feel more comfortable about a statement that is some form of "Science says. . . ."

It would appear that most people have an eclectic approach to interpreting what is reality that goes like this:

> In a democracy everybody's equal . . . right? Well, not really, but any person can be as good as anybody else. Some things may be good for "the people," but *I* decide whether they're good for me. I believe in God . . . I'm a religious person, but I'm no fanatic. Religion has some truth, but not all truth. I believe in science, too, but those guys can go too far sometimes. Science has helped us a lot, but *I* decide what I'll believe and what I'll do. Scientists

---
[2] Hsu, Francis L. K., "A Cholera Epidemic in a Chinese Town," Case 5 in Paul Benjamin (Ed.), *Health, Culture and Community*. New York: Russell Sage Foundation, 1955. pg. 149.

seem to contradict each other a lot. I'd feel better if they could agree . . . but, then, they might get too powerful. There are so many ways to believe . . . a person's just got to decide for himself.

WE KNOW MORE . . . THERE'S MUCH MORE TO KNOW. Most people have some sense of the fact that we know more than perhaps has ever been known. This brings the companion realization that there is more to know than ever before. Put in personal terms, "Doc Bunyan knows more than any doctor did fifty years ago, but there's also so much that he could know but doesn't." We must trust the physician and the teacher, but we also know that they are individuals. Individual human beings, whatever their professional training, have human limitations.

. . . AND NEW DISCOVERIES CAN MEAN DANGER, TOO. Medical science has compiled an impressive record of eliminating or abating certain causes of premature death, in reducing symptoms, and in making it possible for people with disabilities to live a fuller, longer life. Education, with a scientific base, has attempted the difficult task of becoming universal in a culture without some of the values placed on work and sacrifice that most favor educational success . . . and has had rather marked success. Techniques of conditioning, those with the most capacity for achieving desired behavior, have not been used much. We still have and use the derogatory term "brainwashing" for this general approach. Those who believe in God in an orthodox Christian way accept the fact that God could destroy us as a culture. This ultimate power attracts some people, but certainly turns others away. In a somewhat like fashion, science, including medical science, could destroy us, and education, using certain techniques, could change us mightily. Each could have this power, however, only with the faith and allegiance of the populace. So, it seems that the culture considers a certain amount of skepticism about the influence of science and education as healthy.

HEALTH EDUCATION AS PREVENTION. In educational perspective, health education can be seen either as primarily general education or as primarily practical, utilitarian learning. In medical perspective, health education usually is seen as part of prevention, be it primary, secondary, or tertiary. This placing fairly quickly puts it in trouble with the scientific base for medicine. Why? Because, though it can be proved scientifically that something did not happen (Lola did not get tetanus, Ken did not develop any dental caries in six months, Maude did not use angry words when her little brother broke her favorite record album), it is very difficult to prove that it would have happened except for some preventively oriented education. First, there must be some assumption about how likely it is to happen to the individual (Lola, Ken Maude), and then some assumption about the influence of education over, above, or along with other possible influences.

For further example, if we assume that everyone has the potential for becoming an alcoholic, then in this culture 93%-95% of alcoholism is prevented, i.e., does not develop. If we have some basis for assuming that only, say, 20% of the population could become alcoholic, then actual prevention is not as good. If only 7% could be alcoholics and all of them are alcoholics, then our efforts at primary prevention have not worked. If we assume, however, that it can be prevented, how do we decide . . . or better, scientifically determine the exact influence of education in competition with other influences? What shall we call education and what non-education? It might be relatively easy to design a specific educational program, like those in the federally initiated Alcohol Safety Action Projects in the early 1970's, where one can show that a certain group had this experience and another group clearly did not. However, from the viewpoint of pure science, a finding that those in the program displayed less undesirable behavior (got less drunk, drove less after drinking . . .) would be significant only if the composition can be determined, in some gross way, but, outside of strict institutions, there is no way of guaranteeing that the groups have other comparable experiences. We just have to assume they do if we are going to respect the findings.

A CONTINUUM FOR IDEAL EDUCATION. Using alcohol education as an example of a potential force in prevention of various forms of dysfunction, education can be seen from the general to the very utilitarian. An example of this notion is the instrument developed for an early 1970's research project. It is entitled "How Should We Be Educating About Different Substances That Modify Mood and Behavior?" [3] (alcohol being one). The plate below is the cover sheet for the study. It gives the context for judgment and the directions:

DIRECTIONS
There is a range of philosophy that can be the basis for any attempts to educate about use, non-use and misuse of substances that modify mood and behavior.

At one extreme is a philosophy based on the premise that each individual must assess for himself whether use of a substance will be a helpful means of adaptation or a threat to later functioning; the essential controls to avoid abuses are personal controls; education should be as open and unbiased as possible. In short: THE INDIVIDUAL IS CAPABLE OF AVOIDING OR SOLVING HIS OWN PROBLEMS.

---

[3] Russell, Robert D., "Evaluation of 'Ideal' Statements of Educational Philosophy and Goals for Four Mood Modifying Substances in Ecological Perspective," Summer Research Project, College of Education, Southern Illinois University at Carbondale, 1972.

At the other extreme is a philosophy based on the premise that some individual use of substances causes a variety of social problems; the essential controls to protect society must be social controls; education must help to identify problems and individuals who have them, must be part of a program to retrain and recondition abusers, and must, finally, be a major factor in preventing alcohol and drug problems. In short: THE INDIVIDUAL CANNOT AVOID OR SOLVE HIS OWN PROBLEMS AND MUST HAVE HELP FROM SOCIETY.

A middle group philosophy is one that respects individual's rights to choose use or non-use, but also focuses on social problems resulting from unwise choices; controls should be both personal and social (which allow some problems and, at the same time, unnecessarily restrict some people); education should help the individual make decisions, but ultimately tends to focus on problems, thus seeming to discourage most use. In short: THE INDIVIDUAL CAN AVOID OR SOLVE SOME OF HIS OWN PROBLEMS BUT NEEDS SOCIETY'S HELP WITH SOME.

The ideal philosophy for educating young people (ages 12-20) must be some place along a continuum connecting the two extremes— but the ideal may be different for different substances. You are invited to make a judgment of the ideal for each of four substances that modify mood and behavior—alcohol, heroin, LSD, and marijuana. Please read the statements of educational philosophy and then the three sets of representative objectives that a teacher having each philosophy would try to accomplish. Then detach the Response Sheet from the back of the instrument and place it under the words Ideal Basis for Education. Mark the continuum line on the Response Sheet so that it compares to your judgment as to the ideal for each substance. The closer your mark is to a vertical line the more you also favor the philosophy on the other side of the line, despite choosing one of the three philosophies as the most appropriate. You can mark anywhere on the line, except on the two verticals . . . but make only one mark.

Example: ✔ or ——X————— / —— or ✔ or ✔ / —— or X——

After the directions came four pages, exactly alike in format and phrased as nearly alike as possible, considering some real differences in effects and usage and legality among the four substances being probed. Each sheet has three columns in parallel. The three portions are supposed to represent a theoretical column. The three segments are labeled PERSONAL (that roughly agrees with the health education as general education perspective), MIDDLE (some eclectic combination of the two extremes) and SOCIAL (that has a utilitarian concern for specific behaviors and non-behaviors). Each is introduced with a brief statement of basic philosophy. Those for Alcohol are representative of the other three.

PERSONAL

PHILOSOPHY: Alcohol, for many people, is an effective means of adapting to certain life situations and personal needs; for other people, it is a threat to functioning and should be avoided.

Each individual has to discover whether he can or wants to have alcohol as part of his positive life style.

Education can help with this discovery process, but many other factors are more important.

OBJECTIVES: PERSONAL

1. To develop examples of alcohol's positive use as a means by which some people adapt to certain life situations and personal needs.

2. To compare and contrast *use* that looks more like a threat to the drinker and society.

3. To identify some other means of adapting that could be used in place of alcohol—if the consequences of its use become a threat to an individual.

MIDDLE

PHILOSOPHY: Alcohol, though it is used by some people without apparent harm, causes many personal and social problems.

Society helps protect itself and its citizens from more problems by educating young people to know and avoid uses of alcohol that result in problems.

OBJECTIVES: MIDDLE

1. To compare and contrast styles of drinking and drinking incidents that seem harmless with those that seem to be problems.

2. To develop examples of problems created by alcohol—for the individual, for others and for society.

3. To identify solutions to alcohol problems—and ways of avoiding such.

SOCIAL

PHILOSOPHY: Alcohol use results in many serious social problems, and education must be part of a social identification of those who are likely to have problems and part of a program to retrain those toward better functioning. If education is successful, there are no alcohol problems.

OBJECTIVES: SOCIAL

1. To identify the total range of alcohol related problems and types of persons and situations involved.

2. To develop solutions to alcohol problems and commitments on the part of learners to use these solutions—in their own lives and in society.

3. To prevent further problems stemming from man and alcohol.

Although the research has not been completed, certain important general observations can be made. The response sheets gathered thus far indicate that for alcohol, at least 20% of any respondent group, teachers or students, are in each segment of the continuum. In other words, there is no apparent agreement on what the ideal basis for health education should be . . . and therefore, presumably on what its accomplishments should be.

A REVIEW. What has been said thus far? Medicine and education both are oriented to helping humans function better, and both have a base in science as a way of knowing and as a basis for action. Both have a certain amount of authority in the culture . . . and therefore are both respected and resisted.

Both involve content and process. In education there is something to be taught and some way of teaching. In medicine there is knowledge of what observed symptoms might represent and some way of eliminating the cause of these symptoms. In education there is the idea, currently popular among professional educators, that learning is more important than teaching. In medicine there always has been the notion that the body heals itself and the best medicine is that which simply helps the body's own processes.

Both medicine and education have tremendous potential for human good—for improving the function of people of all ages. This potential can be realized as each is practiced by good men and women—conscientious, unselfish, hard-working, sacrificing, intelligent, adaptable people. If practitioners exhibit characteristics other than these, their effectiveness tends to decline and the potential for harm to the culture increases.

PUBLIC-PRIVATE . . . RIGHT-PRIVILEGE. Originally in the American colonies and the new U.S.A., both education and medicine were private enterprises. Parents, or the larger community, taught children, and, if more formal education was desired, parents had to pay for it. Parents, or the larger community, treated incidents of ill-health, and, if trained assistance seemed necessary, it had to be paid for, in some way. Then it was decided that a democracy with emerging adult suffrage must have universal education, and so a conglomerate system of tax-supported schools arose. Education was public and the right and responsibility of every citizen. Because schools were largely funded by local communities, each community had the quality of schools it wished to support. This really was taking the private principle only a step into the local community. Today, there are continuous efforts to diminish the differences in money spent on schools in proximate districts.

TEACHERS AND PHYSICIANS AS PROFESSIONALS. Education, however, was to be for all, so a great many teachers were required. Thus, if teaching was to be a profession, it was destined to be a large profession, serving in states and school districts with a diversity of standards. Therefore, because of numbers and various expectations, it is a profession with a wide range of standards.

The culture decided that education should be tax-supported, but did not make such a decision for medical care. Thus, it was to be privately arranged and paid for. The physician was accorded more status and honor because the profession was associated with that important difference between life and death. The ethic of Hippocrates, the protoιype doctor, called for an apprenticeship system of education. So medical schools remained fairly small and difficult-to-get-into and quality continued high.

CHANGING VIEWS ABOUT MEDICAL CARE. We now are in a time of considering the merits and the costs of making high quality medical care available to all, regardless of ability to pay. The goal of quality medical care for all who need it is a beautiful one . . . in the abstract . . . but the costs of such a change cannot be easily brushed aside. The taxation for such a system, whether directly governmental or via subsidizing insurance carriers, will be horrendous as our brief experience with Medicare and Medicaid suggests. The absolute need for more physicians (or for some people to do what physicians have formerly done . . . however it is worked out) will require money for school, faculty, facilities, and student expenses. Indeed, it is a cost! It is clear that the delivery of medical and health care services is in transition to something, yet there is no full agreement as to what that will ultimately be. Whether it will be more or less scientific . . . more or less people oriented . . . more or less authoritative . . . these answers can come only in the future.

A SUMMARY.
- In this culture medicine and education are dominated more by scientific than by religious thinking.
- In medicine and education, the mandatory safeguards in human research preclude the kind of experimentation that can be called pure science.
- Science discovers; technology converts such discoveries to practical uses; merchandising makes these widely available.
- Explanations other than scientific explanations for happenings are most commonly Fate, Luck, Circumstances.
- Non-scientific thinking is believed because it often comes from persons an individual knows and trusts.
- Some Americans are somewhat skeptical of both religious and scientific truth.

Chapter VI

Attitudes and Other Affectors of Behavior

"Health is really a dumb class . . . I mean, the things we cover are all things we know about . . . everything's so obvious . . . No, I don't do very well, but how can you get interested in things you already know about?"

"Health is the kind of class I really like . . . most of the time we're dealing with things I know something about and am interested in, but then we go on and I learn some more . . . you know, it makes you feel that the things you've already learned are still important, but there's always some more to learn."

"Nobody that I know likes health class . . . there's too much opinion . . . too much of working in groups and listening to stupid people say different things . . . it ought to be more definite . . . there are things to do and not do that'll make you healthy . . . why doesn't the teacher just tell us these things instead of all this involvement?"

"The most important and exciting class I have is health . . . what each of us considers healthy is individual, but we still can learn from each other . . . it's fascinating to hear someone express a view quite different from mine . . . it gives you real experience in changing or keeping your own ideas and in interacting with other kids in relation to some important things."

THE WAY IT SEEMS TO ME. They're all about the same age, are all in the same health class, taught by the same teacher. But their attitudes are not alike and, therefore, the class seems different to each student. Such statements make questions such as—How do students feel about health as a class? . . . about considering the problem of avoiding accidents? . . . about working in groups rather than always sitting as a total class? . . . about dealing with the values as well as the facts in selecting food to eat?—somewhat ridiculous. As noted in an earlier chapter, the behavior of young people does not always reflect what they feel, but, assuming that these statements do represent true feelings, they guarantee that there will be some variety of response to any learning approach attempted in the class. A principle deriving from behavioral research in public health during the 1950's and 1960's holds that behavior is determined by subjective reality rather than objective—by the individual's own motives and beliefs, regardless of whether these correspond to the health educator's notion of reality or the latter's concept of what is good for people.

CLASSROOMS . . . NO PERFECTION. All right, doesn't this virtually eliminate the classroom as a viable site for health education? No, it means only that a class setting can never be a perfect site of learning for all, but it can be for some . . . perhaps even many. The department store tycoon Samuel Wanamaker was once quoted as saying, "I know that at least half of what we spend on advertising is wasted. The trouble is . . . I don't know which half." Some teaching-learning approaches may not be effective with some individuals in a class on a particular day, but it is rarely possible to predict exactly who will learn what and why. Even harder to predict is how each will feel about what has been learned, about the learning activity, and about whether it is worth applying in one's own personal life. Good teachers tend to be those who see such a situation as a challenge in that some success is always possible. Teaching effectiveness is partly a matter of attitude, too.

ATTITUDES THAT ALLOWED SCIENCE. The scientific, and particularly the experimental, study of behavior is a comparatively new enterprise. It could not really develop, of course, until the scientific study of the other, more manipulatable phenomena of the world was established, systematized, reasonably accepted—and some traditions and mores worked out. The premise allowing science was that the natural world was not so sacred that it could not be studied (which did mean manipulation, at times). The study of human behavior was delayed until there was readiness for the relative acceptance of scientific findings as being more helpful than dangerous. So we gradually reached a cultural point where it seemed appropriate to systematically observe human behavior, have human beings take certain tests and do certain prescribed tasks . . . even to have human subjects volunteer to participate in certain experiments.

CAREFUL WITH HUMAN SUBJECTS! All proposals for research that involve human subjects in any way must be screened to determine that there is no potential physical, mental, emotional, even spiritual harm forthcoming for the subjects. I am certain that this is a virtually universal pre-research procedure in this culture.

SCIENTISTS' CRITICISM OF ONE ANOTHER. Science could progress if non-scientists would let up the opposing pressure; scientists certainly are united in relation to the scientific enterprise . . . right? Wrong! Science is basically a method—studying phenomena systematically, setting hypotheses, retesting—but once a particular science is established and gains an amount of recognition, it exhibits some tendency to be critical of some other areas. The criticism tends to focus on methodology, disparaging study design, type and number of subjects, location, time span and lack of control of other variables. These criticisms have value in keeping the quality of scientific endeavor high, but, practically speaking, they also hinder the development of new scientific fields, particularly in the behavioral sciences that directly or indirectly relate to humans.

Since the development of psychiatry and clinical psychology, there has been conflict between scientists about the study of inner being. Some feel that this is an area about which we are relatively ignorant and one that will give forth tremendously important new understanding in the future. Established objective techniques do not apply. How objective can you be if you use essentially subjective techniques for gathering data? The counter to this sounds like, "The essence of science is the systematic study of reality: if reality does not lend itself to investigation by present techniques, then new ones will have to be developed."

THE MAJOR POINTS, then, are (1) that the scientific study of human motives and behavior is of relatively recent origin; (2) that most of what we know comes from systematic observation, from questionnaires and other requests for personal responses; and (3) that true experiments involving human behavior are relatively rare because of our concern for the rights of individuals who would be subjects. Most such experiments (a) have small samples, (b) are done in institutions (hospitals, prisons, schools), (c) cannot control all affecting variables, and (d) often involve some related but safer task than that for which data are desired. Science is a new way of knowing, and the culture holds to other values more strongly than "letting science off the tether" in knowing about human beings. Nevertheless, we do know much more about how and why people function than before the social and behavioral sciences were decanted.

MOTIVES AND BEHAVIOR. Two important concepts that need to be developed as means of understanding behavior are those of motives and attitudes.

- Motives are the basic predispositions to strive toward certain general goals . . . for instance, Jenny wants to be the leader of the gang of kids in her neighborhood, and that leads her to stand up to a strong person who threatens her leadership of the gang.

- Elmer's attitude toward teachers is generally positive because he feels that they are instrumental in his being a good student; his attitude toward television is mildly negative because, though he recognizes there are some educational programs shown, in general television seduces him away from his studies.

- **Sheri** has a fairly strong negative attitude toward planned parenthood and zero population growth because she feels that they generally disparage her strong desire to marry and have a large family.

DISCOVERING ATTITUDES. Attitudes are a component of the goal of most health education experiences. But attitudes also affect how and what each student will learn. How, then, does a teacher (or a researcher) discover what attitudes learners have? In basically three ways:

(1) By asking directly (verbal or written to select the most appropriate answer response)

- How do you feel about smoking?

(2) By asking indirectly

- If a person sitting next to you in a bus was smoking and offered you a cigarette, what would you say and do?

(3) By inferring from observed behavior

- When a person sitting near Maggie starts to smoke she begins to appear very uncomfortable and will move to another seat if she can; she refuses proffered cigarettes with very minimal courtesy.

Basically, the same principles apply in discovering motives. The reader may wish to create examples of each.

Health-related behavior has one of two basic orientations, though in real life these certainly do not exist as separate, dichotomous categories; many actions are some mixture of each.

(1) Behavior when one is ill, injured, incapacitated, or otherwise in poor health

(2) Behavior to prevent such dysfunctioning states from occurring

In addition, health often finally culminates in urging

(a) A behavior . . . doing something such as

- Brushing teeth . . . drinking fruit juice . . . helping a younger person acquire a new skill . . . working to promote a worthy cause, such as a cleaner environment and

(b) A non-behavior . . . not doing something

- Not eating candy excessively . . . not being an isolate . . . not burning old dry leaves

PETER'S ATTITUDES AND MOTIVES. Let's observe a behavioral example of attitudes and motives that could be behind a note a school nurse, teacher, principal, or attendance officer might receive: "Please excuse Peter's absence from school on Monday and Tuesday. He had a sore throat and was under a doctor's care."

Peter, age 14, wakes up Monday morning and, as he swallows, becomes aware that his throat is sore. A sore throat is not usual for him; it is irritating and uncomfortable, so he quickly develops a motive. His goal is to get rid of the pain in his throat. He has a favorable attitude toward cool water as a cure and he drinks some. It gives no lasting relief. He has a favorable attitude toward gargling with salt and soda as a cure. He does this, but it gives no lasting relief. His attitudes toward these two practices are still positive, but strength of his attitude has diminished because neither seem helpful. What does he do now?

Peter has some conflicts to resolve. He has positive attitudes toward both school and medical care. He has no real objection either to going to school or going to his family doctor. Whichever he does will be in place of the other. He is motivated to go to school, but he is also motivated by the desire to play in an important basketball game on Thursday. So he elects to share the decision-making with his parents. If they (even one of them) would have "pooh-poohed" the potential seriousness of the pain, had given him some throat lozenges and told him to go to school, he probably would have done so. However, his mother takes his temperature and finds it over two degrees above normal; both his parents agree that he should go to the physician instead of school, and his father reinforces this with the observation, "If you get it treated today you should be well and in good shape to play your best basketball on Thursday." Peter's attitude toward getting medical care is positive, and with the external support of his parents toward the motive of getting well faster with medical care, he misses school and receives treatment and rests at home instead.

His attitude toward prompt medical care is probably reinforced if his throat does well by Thursday, and he is able to play in the game . . . because the action on Monday seems related to his strong motive, achieved on Thursday. (Of course, for this reinforcement to be maximal, he must have a minimum of feeling, "I'd have felt just as good if I hadn't wasted all that time with the doctor.")

If, on the other hand, that wait at the doctor's office seemed interminable, the physician wasn't friendly, the injection was painful, and he still felt lousy on Thursday, his attitude toward the chosen course of action is less apt to be positive. Or if his missing basketball practice Monday and Tuesday resulted in his being replaced on the starting five and in his playing very little, then his motive was not satisfied by the action and therefore the attitude toward it as a future thing to do is less prone to be positive.

IS THE ABOVE EXAMPLE REALISTIC? Actual living, of course, is much more complex than this example suggests, but have you ever tried describing all the possible attitudes, motives and behavior interacting in even such a thin slice of life as the foregoing? It seems that however much you write down, there still is more that could be said . . . or the effects could have been thus, instead, or . . . and . . . because. . . .

COGNITIVE DISSONANCE. In the first chapter, if you remember, attitudes and behavior were described in interaction with knowledge. We can reintroduce this cerebral factor in acknowledging and briefly describing the phenomenon of cognitive dissonance.[1] Cognitive dissonance is the internal discomfort that arises in individuals when they know something they should or should not do, but are urged to behave counter to this knowledge. Since attitude is the other factor in this triumvirate, it may throw the balance one way or the other. A fundamental importance of cognitive dissonance is that the state is uncomfortable for most individuals . . . even painful for some. The hope behind much health education is that if a learner gains and internalizes new information (which becomes knowledge for her/him) that suggests that a present form of behavior is not a contributor to good health, the person will resolve the dissonance by bringing behavior in line with knowledge. Example: If Sarah learns and comes to know how automobile seatbelts prevent sudden, unexpected body movement in the car and that their use is actually correlated with fewer injuries and deaths than for folk not wearing belts in comparable accidents, she may increase the frequency of her buckling up (even become a regular). This is more likely if she has an attitude toward descriptions of past accidents like, "That could happen to me, too." If this occurs, her dissonance is reduced or eliminated, and a safer behavior has been motivated by knowledge of possible consequences.

However, if her attitudes (including, "That wouldn't happen to me") do not push her to use of belts, then the dissonance remains and still cries to be reduced. The less desirable result (from the viewpoint of traditional health education) is that she "turns off" learning about the value of belts, forgets what she learns, and/or searches for other information that tells of deaths and injuries that have occurred because the victim was buckled in tightly. Then the attitude, "Well, I wouldn't want that to happen to me" helps reduce the dissonance, and there seems to be more consistency between what she knows and what she does.

LEGISLATED OR COMPELLED BEHAVIOR. Since this latter-described result seems too frequent for some advocates of more accident prevention, some state legislatures now are considering legislation that, in effect, would try to reduce the dissonance of car occupants by an opposite strategy. Rather than trying to get desired behavior from knowledge, proposed laws would make it illegal not to have a seat belt

---

[1] Festinger, Leon, *A Theory of Cognitive Dissonance.* Evanston, Illinois: Row, Peterson & Co., 1957. Ch. 1.

fastened when driving or riding. People then obeying the law would be doing something they do not believe in. So to reduce the dissonance they will come to believe and feel that what they are doing is a good and potentially helpful, rewarding behavior. Just as people can and do justify potentially dangerous behavior, people can and do justify safer behavior. In simple terms, we like to feel and have evidence for the fact that what we're doing is good, healthful, or right.

Suffice it to say, briefly, that some people, including some of the young, do not seem to suffer much from cognitive dissonance. Such seem blithely capable of admitting they know they should do this or that . . . and should not do that and this . . . and still behave contrary to what they know without apparent discomfort. Perhaps all theories of human behavior can only describe a central tendency. Perhaps no principle accurately describes all individuals at all times. The epitome of a qualified statement!

SUSCEPTIBILITY, SERIOUSNESS, AND MEANS OF PREVENTION OR CONTROL. The major generalizations about preventive behavior—why people do or do not take actions that prevent certain departures from full health—blossomed from the work and analysis of several behavioral scientists associated with the Behavior Studies Section of the U.S. Public Health Service in the late 1950's and early 1960's. Rosenstock [2] and Hochbaum [3] probably deserve the major credit for the following model:

". . . an individual's motivation in relation to any particular health issue is determined largely by three kinds of beliefs:

1. the extent to which he sees it as a health problem with high probability of affecting him personally

2. the extent to which she believes the problem would have serious consequences for her if it *did* involve her

3. the extent to which she believes some *reasonable* course of action open to her would be effective in reducing the threat"

Thus, beliefs about susceptibility, seriousness, and means to prevent or control are determiners of action or inaction: a person lacking one or more becomes less likely to take action.

An example: four teenage girls are anticipating the ski season and definitely are "thinking snow," but they seem to vary in their response to a health-related message. They all hear that they should

2 Rosenstock, Irwin M., "What Research in Motivation Suggests for Public Health," *American Journal of Public Health.* 50: 298, March 1960. See also Rosenstock's entry in *The Health Belief Model and Personal Health Behavior,* Marshall H. Becker, guest editor. *Health Education Monographs,* 2, Winter 1974.

3 Hochbaum, Godfrey M., *Health Behavior.* Belmont, California: Wadsworth Publishing Co., Inc., 1970. pp. 56-57.

begin to do some prescribed exercises daily to strengthen knees and ankles and, in general, the muscles of the legs to prevent injuries and sore legs during the early part of the season.

- Marian does the exercises because she recognizes soreness and injuries as problems to avoid that could affect her; she also feels that they could happen to her and that these exercises are a reasonable, possibly effective preventive measure.

- Melody does not do the exercises because she just doesn't believe soreness or injury will happen to her.

- Maribeth does not do the exercises because, although she thinks it could happen to her, she doubts that anything of this nature would be serious enough to warrant this time and energy for exercises.

- Meg does not do the exercises because, although she knows injury and soreness are serious and feels that they could happen to her, she just doesn't believe exercises are a realistic prevention; she believes that the only way to strengthen yourself is just to ski.

So only one young woman follows the preventive course and three do not—but each for a different reason.

CONFLICT . . . INCONSISTENCY. Two other principles derived from the experiments and other systematic studies of health-related behavior seem worth noting. The first: an individual's motives and beliefs in regard to various courses of action often are in conflict with one another; actual behavior results from some resolution of the conflict. The stronger motive generally will determine behavior, and for many people, health motives are not as strong as many other imperatives to action. The second: health-related motives may not always result in appropriate health behavior . . . and health-related behavior may result from motives that are not oriented to health. Two examples of this second statement:

- Meredith feels he would be better off if he lost twenty pounds, so he gets some "uppers" from some friends making the drug scene, gets high and stays high for four weekends in a row, resulting in the loss of twenty pounds—a health-related motive, but extreme and dangerous as a behavior.

- On the other hand, Thad decides that the price of meat is too high so he cuts down to having meat only three or four days a week, still well within body needs and potentially more healthful from a fat content perspective—a better state of health resulting from an economic motive.

ORIENTATIONS—PERSONAL AND SOCIAL. The culture of the U.S.A. today is one of many competing influences. Each individual obviously has a unique set of life experiences, not shared in their entirety by any other fellow human. On the more general level, however, some persons and groups are exposed to more of one influence than others, and each individual also selects either a balance of orientations or an orientation that predominates in developing motives. And these, of course, eventually produce behavior.

Some people have a predominantly personal orientation, and for these, most strong motives are aligned with self-betterment.

- Jane rarely drives after consuming alcoholic drinks because she doesn't want to risk an accident in which she might be killed or maimed, personally . . . she gives blood at the blood bank so that she will be eligible for blood should she ever need a transfusion . . . she eats vegetables because their vitamin-mineral content should benefit her health. . . .

Others have strong social orientations, with strong motives based on the good of society or of some particular others.

- Jim rarely drives after consuming alcoholic drinks because he realizes that this can make him dangerous to others on the road, possibly hurting or killing innocent people . . . he gives blood at the blood bank because each pint may help save someone else's life . . . he eats vegetables because his wife serves them and he doesn't want to get into a hassle with her. . . .

Some homes and sub-cultures emphasize the personal orientation more . . . others emphasize the social or group motives. Maturity, in this culture, is usually seen as having some balance of both. However, any health-related message designed to stimulate motives for behavior that has a predominantly personal orientation will most likely be accepted by learners with the same way of thinking and be ignored by those with more social orientation. And vice versa.

YOU'LL APPRECIATE IT LATER. Another crucial orientation for many health-related decisions is the future. Most small children and individuals with limited basic intelligence have truncated senses of the future. They do not respond appropriately to admonitions to "do this now in order to prevent that . . . later." Growing and developing normally extends and makes more real this sense of the future. It is generally easier to get acceptance of smoking as dangerous because of possible lung cancer or emphysema forty or so years in the future in a senior high class than in a junior high group. Acceptance is likely to be greater among the better students, and in a school with mostly upper income, middle class youngsters. Health professionals, including health educators, tend to have considerable sense of the future. It is just as important to recognize that many learners in health do not naturally have such an orientation. Though health education may help to develop such an orientation, some other motives should be on deck for those more present-oriented.

One piquant deviation from the norm just exposited is that somewhat individualistic yet also somewhat conforming group attitude held by a segment of today's youth. They are striving to develop a life-style without some of the short-comings they perceive in the society. On the one hand, there is a strong preference for the present rather than the future that would, for instance, legitimize the use of drugs for a present potential high rather than non-use in order to avoid some possible future difficulties. On the other hand, there may be an opposition to the present construction of an electric power plant because of the environmental insults that may accrue in the future. The best generalization, I suppose, is the counter attitude in relation to issues for which the general culture thinks of the future; this group favors the present . . . for others, it is future over the present. Obviously, their willingness to relate to education based on an opposite orientation tends to be minimal.

PAIN: SAVOR OR AVOID? Another orientative attitude that deserves at least a mention in any health discussion is that toward pain.

One polar attitude (probably not held by many Americans today— but some) would view pain as a basically healthy experience, both as an indication of some confrontation with the body or mind and as something to experience as a means of growth. The opposite polar view sees pain as wholly undesirable; health behavior always is that which avoids, reduces or eliminates pain. Some people, then, are motivated strongly to avoid pain. What they do and do not do stems from projections about potential pain. Let's take an example of a person with a different attitude. Russ was a middle teenager on a football team I was coaching who had an unusual willingness to hurl himself into blockers in order to spoil a play or to try for a tackle despite the pounding and stomping it might entail. His adopted father told me that, as a small boy, he apparently got genuine pleasure out of riding his scooter down a fairly steep hill and deliberately crashing it into a tree. Avoidance of pain just did not seem to be one of his strong motives.

A contemporary and famous example of willingness to endure pain for fame and fortune is Joe Namath, quarterback for the New York Jets during the late 1960's and early 1970's. A health educator with a strong orientation to the future and away from pain would deplore as unhealthy Mr. Namath's willingness to risk further injury for present goals. Joe, probably, would like to have his options other than they are (i.e., to have all strong, original, unoperated-upon joints), but this not being possible, he risks and hurts in order to achieve his goals.

TEACHERS' ATTITUDES. The implications of these truths about attitudes and motives for health teachers are several. Each teacher will develop and display some position on health-related behavior. Some teachers' classroom attitudes will be identical with their own personal attitudes. Other teachers will evidence some amount of inconsistency, expressing certain personal attitudes and then appearing not to have attitudes on other issues, mainly because how they really feel is different from how they think they should feel. Health teachers may demonstrate extreme liberal attitudes, leaning toward a dynamic duo of statements such as the following:

"Any behavior may be healthy for a particular individual . . . depending on his or her personal values."

"Even though ———— may be dangerous (not be good) for most people, it might be all right for a particular individual . . . you never know until you try it."

Other health teachers might demonstrate extremely conservative attitudes. The baseline attitudes of these conservative leaders would sound thusly: "There are certain ways of thinking and behaving that are healthy, and others that are not . . . it is my task to get students to think and feel and act as they should."

"We know what behaviors involve risking good health . . . health education generally should encourage learners not to take risks . . . and to understand why."

Then, of course, there are those (perhaps a majority?) who mount some personal and/or pedagogical compromises that have this flavor:

"Each person has to decide for herself or himself whether the pleasures and values of smoking cigarettes and drinking alcoholic beverages override the risks, but using heroin or sopors is just too dangerous . . . it would be foolish to try these."

"Each person has to make up her or his own mind what social causes to support and what social causes to oppose, but sitting in on the construction site of a nuclear power plant is going too far . . . is unhealthy social behavior."

HEALTH BEHAVIOR NOT IN THE CLASSROOM. As was indicated earlier, attitudes are generally evaluated by observing behavior. Oh, it can be argued that Joe can believe one thing and do another . . . for instance, Joe believes in protecting himself against infections, but he did cut himself while working on his car last Saturday afternoon, and he didn't even wash it until after he finished the job in the evening. Maybe it is true that Joe believes one thing and does another, but the actual behavior suggests that however strong his attitudes toward protecting himself from infections may be, they are less strong than those toward going on with the job, despite an injury. In terms of infection, he just has to have some attitude of "It won't happen to me" that overpowers the attitude pleading for caution and prompt care. This all congeals into the generalization that most health-related behaviors cannot be observed in the health class. The teacher can observe and evaluate academic behavior . . . and classroom social behavior . . . and classroom evidences of emotional expression and control, and can ask for verbal or written recalls or predictions of behavior. But the teacher cannot know directly whether:

- Joe does or does not disinfect cuts promptly.

- Shirley does or does not smoke pot, and how often and how much.

- Benedict does or does not display hostility toward others when driving at night.

- Alyce does or does not overdo the use of home remedies for real or imagined ills.

What is learned in the classroom must be carried over by each learner to that situation where the knowledge and the attitude interact with motives and where behavior or non-behavior results. Obviously, such situations are often quite unlike classroom experiences.

- The evaluation of some learning in a 7th grade class on refusing to start smoking involved writing, on Wednesday, a simulation of a weekend situation (party or otherwise) and describing how an individual could skillfully and without embarrassment refuse an offer of a cigarette. Jayne's response was imaginative, thorough and accurate; she earned a maximum number of points on this test item, but the test was not returned by Friday. On Saturday evening, as she was putting the finishing touches on her hair, she mused, before her mirror at 6:30 p.m., about what she might do and not do, how she might react to various happenings at the party to which she was going. Here she was almost as rational as on her exam question, but later in the evening, with a small group of girls under a tree in the party's back yard, she did not react according to her response on the exam.

SOME CARRY-OVER HYPOTHESES. Somehow the carry-over was eroded. Are there ways to prevent this from happening? Nothing proven, but consider some hypotheses based on behavioral science. First, the positive: the type of evaluation was probably as close to reality as possible. The task was a written simulation of real life, with the writer having to set the situation and reactions. This certainly would theoretically be better reinforcement of learning than a true-false question such as, Do women smokers develop heart diseases as frequently as men? False is the correct answer, but it gives you no clue as to how much more the student knows, doesn't know, or knows in part. One shortcoming, from the behavioral perspective, is that the exam was given on Wednesday, a maximum distance from a past weekend and from an upcoming one, and probably more social opportunities to light up. This could have been remedied, even exploited, if the exam had been returned and discussed with some thoroughness on Friday . . . a revisiting . . . a reinforcement.

For maximum impact on behavior, in theory, the learner must really give her/his attention to the learning situation. There should be reinforcement of major points to be learned, and the reinforcement should increasingly make the learner apply the ideas, facts, concepts to be learned in new situations that are close to the learner's real life. Some research suggests that if a learner makes some sort of tangible commitment to actually do or not do something, there is more likelihood of the actual behavior being consistent. Finally, the closer all of this classroom activity occurs to actual situations of like decisions, the less likely forgetting and other counter-learnings are to interfere. Finally, of course, actual results are powerful influencers. If Jayne did all of the wrong things, exposed herself blatantly to pregnancy and still did not become pregnant, the learning is a mixed bag. And future behavior is not really predictable.

BE AFRAID. Some research suggests that fear (a beguiling, seductive motive that one is often tempted to encourage) may be an effective means to get attention, but is not a good way of encouraging positive behavior.[4] Fear tends to focus on what learners should not do, which often gives no direct clue as to what to do instead . . . and why.

Another important realization for the health educator is that messages and learning experiences designed to heighten fear of a particular behavior (the dangers of unprescribed barbiturate use, for example) may make it seem very attractive to certain youngsters hungry to try something most people are afraid of.

BEHAVIOR MODIFICATION. Now, no chapter on attitudes, motives, and behavior would be respectable at this date without some description and analysis of behavior modification. Originated philosophically, and to an extent empirically, by B. F. Skinner, Harvard psychologist, behavior modification is based on a rather mechanistic view of human action and inaction. It denies any supernatural influences and posits that the behavior of most individuals is not really determined by free will or personal decisions, but by social and cultural conditioning. We all are being programmed to respond in certain predictable ways, but, uncontrolled, this programming produces much undesirable behavior. So why not systematically program people so that they enjoy behaving in ways that are satisfying to them and are non-harmful, even helpful to others? The central strategy is to reward desired behavior, as immediately as possible, and to ignore undesired behavior. Punishment is

---

[4] Russell, Robert D. and Robbins, Paul, "Health Education and the Use of Fear: A New Look," *Journal of School Health.* 34: 267-8, June 1964.

considered a potential kind of reward . . . at least it constitutes recognition and attention; positive or negative may not be important to the behavior. The opposite of rewarding, then, is ignoring. As the individual responds to reward, she/he tends to behave in ways that keep rewards coming. Consequently, behavior is repeated and becomes more comfortable than previous ways of acting. If the behavior (or non-behavior) is also intrinsically rewarding, this more lasting motive begins to take over. Then, to reduce any possible dissonance, the person's attitudes move into agreement with behavior. In theory, all data for behavior modification should come from experiments or other forms of empirical analysis. If it is proposed that some group of unfortunate people can be deconditioned from some destructive behavior and re-trained by a reward system to behave in nonharmful ways . . . it is because experiments show this, in fact, does occur.

WE'VE ALWAYS HAD IT. Behavior modification always has had a hallowed place in schools. Take reading, for example; it is the fundamental behavior taught in schools. Accurate, expressive good reading is rewarded extrinsically at first, until it becomes obvious how useful reading is to accomplish many other tasks . . . and how rewarding it is in and of itself. The efficient reader is rewarded. The poor reader is not. Modern approaches to teaching those with reading difficulties typically are based on giving rewards for progress . . . and withholding the punishments that tend to accrue to those who do not read normally.

HOW MUCH IS HEALTHY? The philosophical value question as to how much behavior modification belongs in health education remains unresolved for the total profession. In a sense, behavior modification is anti-intellectual. It basically denies that reasoning or personal decisions based on weighing alternatives ever is a free process and affirms that its practice produces too many bad decisions. Get people to behave the way they should, and life will be happier for all—becomes the substitute goal. Its practice depends on clear agreement on what the behavioral goal is and then perhaps fierce persistence in seeing that this behavior is rewarded and does begin to predominate.

DIFFICULTIES TEACHERS HAVE. Health education certainly is based on behavior, but it can also deal with attitudes and motives that influence. And, in the classroom or semi-structured settings, it is accomplished in large part through vocabulary and increasing familiarity with pertinent verbal symbols. The general behavior science axiom would be to work from where the learner is. With a normally heterogeneous class of twenty-five or more students, it is difficult to find a place where any appreciable number actually are. This is a fundamental reason why education is not more effective. I talked recently to a teacher who had tried and then given up on complete individualized instruction that is an obvious answer to ineffectiveness. She said, "One day I looked around and it seemed as if I was the only one doing any work and I was worn to a frazzle . . . and the results didn't seem worth the effort." If all teachers were paragons of service dedicated to learners, more learning might take place. But teachers are human beings also whose interests, time allotments, and energies are shared with people and things other than their students. Computers and other forms of programmed instruction can overcome this shortcoming and can tirelessly and with singleness of purpose help a learner progress from where she/he is to a higher understanding. But only if the learner is motivated. If he/she won't turn the page properly or push the right buttons, the program or the computer mutely and powerlessly waits. Only the human teacher has the capacity to deal with lagging desires to learn.

All teachers must decide . . . or evolve a strategy as to . . . how much to be themselves and how much they need to play the role of good teachers. "This above all, to thine own self be true" is an appetizing aphorism, but can have disastrous effects when the teacher is not a natural, caring, resourceful director of learning. For the benefit of learning, some teachers need to learn to be actors and actresses. Is this bad? How do you answer the question, Who is the best performer . . . the actress who plays essentially herself in similar characters or the one who can play a wide variety of characters and be very convincing? If you favor playacting, you conclude that just oneself by itself may not alone be enough.

SUMMARY

- Differences in the attitudes of individual learners result in different reactions to a health class.

- Americans generally believe in science, but few true experiments with human subjects are allowed . . . evidence of values higher than knowing through science.

- Motives and attitudes, unique basic predispositions within each individual, affect health-related behavior.

- Strongest attitudes are those associated with one or more motives.

- A person's beliefs about her/his susceptibility, the seriousness of a threat, and the nature of the means of prevention or control basically determine how the person behaves.

- Attitudes cannot be easily identified by a teacher because much important health-related behavior occurs away from school.

Chapter VII

Risk-Taking

- One night Margi takes an aspirin . . . the next night she takes a poly-drug trip—a chance combination of uppers and downers.

- One afternoon Charles comes down the stairs in his home two at a time without holding the rail . . . the next afternoon he rides his motorcycle down a steep mountain trail, through a stream and up another steep mountain.

- One evening Ken introduces himself to Barby and decides to strike up a friendship . . . one evening two weeks later he asks her to marry him.

Risk-taking comes in many forms and is exhibited in many degrees. Life itself is a matter of risk-taking, but injury, illness, and crippling often result from taking risks, thus making subsequent life less pleasant and more painful. Premature death fairly frequently results from a risk taken, and death certainly diminishes the quality of life. So I have put the negative first, as a health educator would be expected to, but close on its heels is the positive—the reason for this chapter. A risk is any action for which there is some possibility of failure and some possibility of success. For an individual, however, this has to be translated as some possibility for personal satisfaction, pleasure, or sense of accomplishment, with the alternatives being disappointment, pain (or death), or sense of failure. For any individual who takes a risk freely and willingly, the advantages of succeeding seem equal to, or typically greater than, the price of failure.

HEALTH EDUCATION—ANTI-RISK? Issue by issue, behavior by behavior, health education normally opts against risk-taking. Issue by issue, behavior by behavior, this is logical, sensible, defensible. But in this case, healthy parts do not a healthy whole make. Why? Because many real pleasures, exciting experiences, and true accomplishments result only from taking risks. Consistently cautious behavior can stunt a person's functioning. And stunted functioning is, as a denial of one of our original definitions, not healthy. A motto that I like, and feel applies here is, "Moderation in all things, including moderation."

BETTER: HEALTH-BALANCING RISKS. What this boils down to is that healthy people take certain risks and certain precautions. They balance their risks. But, aye, here's the rub: healthy Americans do not necessarily agree on what risks to take and what risks to avoid. There are risks in all dimensions of life—physical, mental, emotional and social risks. And, of course, any particular behavior may be some unique combination of these dimensions. In addition, the pleasures, experiences and accomplishments potentially accruing are not valued uniformly by people. Part of my individuality is tied up with how I value certain experiences and what I'm willing to risk for them . . . and yours is, too.

Let's go back and consider the three risk-takers who introduced this chapter. Margi's taking an aspirin is a risk most of us would take; oh, there are some vague and unlikely dangers, but the feeling of relief from pain certainly seems worth achieving, at a small risk. But when Margi takes a combination of illicit pills for the potential exciting mental-emotional experience it provides, in spite of the risks of panic, confusion, irrationality, psychotic break and suicide, she becomes a small minority of Americans who consider such a risk a desirable one. When Charles comes down the stairs in his home in the fashion described (something he may have done many times), he takes a certain risk, but not a very severe or serious one, particularly for, say a young man of 17 or 20 years. But when he mounts his cycle and roars it down and up steep mountain trails for the physical challenge and emotional charge this action provides, in spite of the potential for serious injury, disablement and violent death that such a ride entails, he is taking a risk most people would value as not worth it!

When Ken introduces himself to Barby and persists in the getting acquainted conversation, he is running a risk of being turned down or of having her show disinterest in him (a social risk with ego involvement), but most of this culture would judge this as a normal, acceptable risk for a mature person. But when he asks her to marry him after only two weeks of acquaintance because they seem made for each other, most of us probably would label this an unwise risk. We probably would judge that the chances are high that their romantic attraction is the main motivation rather than honest evidence of long-term compatibility. But these are extremes, and as different people rate intermediate risks, they will typically exhibit different values. For instance, how risky is it for Margi to smoke a couple of marijuana "joints" or drink two or three screwdrivers? . . . or for Charles to ride his cycle a couple of miles to a movie? . . . or for Ken to ask Barby to marry him after six months of acquaintance and courtship?

DEATH OR HANDICAP. As suggested earlier, there are risks in every dimension of living. The most obvious physical one is death, and the feelings of strongest avoidance are in people who are enjoying life, and who have no strong belief in any after-life existence, either in a spiritual or a reincarnation sense. However, the situations in which death has occurred for someone encompass almost every conceivable life activity, so people tend to try to avoid the risk of death according to their estimate of the general probabilities and their own personal vulnerability. One further return to an initial example: at 17 Charles runs little risk in coming down the stairs two at a time without holding the handrail. However, if Charles is 67, suffering from gout and recovering from a serious heart attack, he considers this type of descent as much more risky—to be executed only in the face of some more immediate threat to life such as his house being on fire.

Another motive of avoidance is in relation to possible handicap. Because most people value wholeness of body and maximum performance, there is an encouragement to eschew risks that could result in loss of vision, loss of limbs, heart attacks, and other diminishers of function. But like the situation for death, it is virtually impossible to live actively and not run some disability risks. So, again, we judge . . . and not always consistently.

MENTAL RISKING. An example of a mental risk is to have to give evidence that one does not know something one is expected to know. Some teachers conduct classes in a very controlled fashion so that they are always in control and run minimal risks of being asked something they should know but do not know. Other teachers feel that this is a risk worth running in order to achieve more active learning in students. So the risk of being considered "dumb" is one many people do not like to run.

In the emotional realm, embarrassment, disappointment and wounded pride are risks attached to many potential activities. To try out for the lead in a play is risky because only one person will achieve and the others may be disappointed and hurt in the pride center. The greater the competition, the more satisfaction one can feel in achieving, but the greater is the sense of disappointment in the many who tried and failed.

SOCIAL RISKING. This shades, of course, across into the realm of risking social disapproval or rejection. Peer pressure in youth groups is partly a matter of suggestions for behavior by certain designated or self-appointed leaders, coupled with the unwillingness of others in the group to risk disapproval or rejection of counter-proposals by the group. Those who risk tend to be leaders; those who shy away from social risks are generally destined to be followers.

PERSONAL CHOICES AND SOCIAL CONTROLS. As in most facets of behavior, some people are reasonably consistent and predictable in relation to the risks they will take, and some people are not. Some are more prone to risks in certain dimensions, some in others. In general, people are more willing to risk when they feel they have some competence in the area of risk . . . and those who do risk tend to develop more ability, thus reducing the degree of risk. The youngster who risks the dangers of learning to ski may learn to ski so expertly that the risks are much diminished. The risks of being dubbed a novice are also reduced, as are those of feeling personally inferior. But the initial risk has to be run and overcome.

A fascinating aspect of risk-taking, however, is that once society recognizes some activity as risky, it develops some controls and deterrents for those who might take the risk. But in order to keep up the support for such controls (particularly if they require periodic refunding), society, or the control agency, needs losers to the risk threat. For example, campaigns to reduce traffic accidents tend to focus on the numbers and conditions of accidents. Ironically, if accidents are reduced markedly, the social concern for controls diminishes; eventually accidents increase again, examples of carnage are once again evident, and controls are reestablished. This tends to be true not because we are insensitive, but on the seemingly simple premise that as a risk seems to diminish, it can be replaced in our concern by others that now seem more serious.

AFRAID OF RISKING. The general thesis developed thus far is that taking certain risks or too many risks can constitute unhealthy behavior. Now let us consider the opposite—being unwilling to take acceptable risks. Evaluate this example: Some years back I met a man in a southwestern state who ran a health studio. As we became acquainted, he told me about some of the people who worked out regularly at his spa, among whom was a certain nineteen-year-old boy. The man was obviously very proud of him as he showed me some pictures, and the lad surely was one of the most perfectly developed physical specimens I had ever glimpsed. Good looking, muscular, steady of gaze, serious in his weight lifting—he looked to be a picture of perfect health (as we usually judge such . . . by physical appearance). But the man went on to say, "He does have one little idiosyncracy—he won't let anyone touch him, even me. You see, he doesn't want to come in contact with germs, and he thinks people carry germs. So he doesn't want to take any chances . . . and letting people touch him is a chance." This struck me as a tragic example of a young person crippling himself emotionally and socially because he was unwilling to take a risk that is so minor it barely deserves an appellation.

Let's assume we have enough generalizations and need to consider now some specific risks.

INFECTIONS. An elaboration on the example of the preceding story —encountering microorganisms—might be in order. After nearly twenty years of parenting, the following risk is being diminished for me. I sit down in a chair and up into my lap crawls one of my sons, exhibiting the vivid symptoms of the common cold—running nose, sneezing, coughing. I know that if I cuddle him and talk to him at close range, his breathing and probable sneezing on me will expose me beautifully, and

I run the risk of manifesting the same symptoms. But in order to avoid this risk I must run the risk of communicating to this little kid that his Daddy doesn't like him. He cannot yet understand the chain of infection and how I must avoid close contact with anyone who has an infection passed in droplets from the nose and throat. All he knows is that I am rejecting him . . . and he didn't do anything. So during these years I often run this risk—and lose too frequently for respiratory comfort. In general, then, close personal contact with another person involves the risk of respiratory infection. And often this seems a risk worth running.

Another related risk is that of infection through a break in the skin. The epitome of caution in regard to this risk is that of the surgeon who scrubs and washes her/his hands and arms for five full minutes before and then, in addition, wears rubber gloves during even a minor surgery. The epitome of recklessness would be administering no treatment at all to a jagged puncture wound, the result of stepping on a dirty nail. Some people would stand aghast at the risk involved in the latter. Others, from experience, would say, Well, the body seems to be able to combat any infections . . . at least I always seem to heal up all right. Still others might have a regular tetanus toxoid booster as recommended by their physicians, and then be rather cavalier about other possible infections. Each break in the skin, accidentally or purposefully made, carries a risk of infection. Yet different individuals vary greatly in how they deal with such risks.

GAMES, SPORTS, AND ATHLETICS often are arenas of risk. Minor risks are pulled, strained and sore muscles, abrasions, blisters, bumps and bruises. As a sport involves more violent body contact (up to collision sports like football and hockey), the risks of serious injury to the brain or central nervous system, the eyes, the joints and the heart increase. Yet, for many players, the risk factor is one of the reasons for competing. The excitement of risking injury in a number of ways produces an emotional satisfaction that is part of the motive for competition. And our judgments about this have some beguiling ambiguities: I recently watched a championship women's gymnastic meet in which one contestant was going to try a particularly difficult and dangerous conclusion to a vault. She had a spotter because of the danger. She completed the maneuver, but the judges ruled that the spotter had touched her. Consequently, she received such a low score that she dropped from a possible winner to last place. The message seems to be that one who tries too blatantly to avoid risk or injury cannot qualify as a champion. This example highlights the mental-emotional risk of sports also. She wanted to win; she made the decision to try this difficult task to insure that win. On a technical ruling she did not succeed and thus lost everything. Her mind then may replay the choice and cry out, If I had done

. . . instead. . . . . In competition, to the extent that one truly enjoys victory, one is susceptible to the hurting disappointment of losing.

SURVIVAL. Risk is intensified in certain types of competition—things like survival camps and expeditions such as "Outward Bound" and "Underway," where participants must scale cliffs, rappel off rock faces, stay out in the wilderness alone, canoe down rapids, survive off the land. Participants are taught how to perform each activity as safely as possible; most can be learned only by actually doing them, with the risk ever present. Various primitive cultures have had some sort of ritualized rites of passage from childhood into adulthood that often require tremendous physical and emotional risk. However frightening these may be, they typically seem less risky than the social disapproval of failing or refusing to try. If this test is the only way to become a legitimate adult, and this is the only desirable thing to be, then whatever risks are entailed are worth running. This culture of ours is much more safety and anti-pain oriented and has no such official rites. However, it is likely that we have in our population some young men and women who are psychologically attuned to this "doing something brave to prove yourself." Even when they are not compelled, they seem unable to advance into adulthood without attempting some risky feat. Such young people race motorcycles or snowmobiles, climb unsurmountable mountains, ski-jump and other potentially dangerous activities, including, unfortunately, sometimes racing automobiles on public highways.

Perhaps one of the most colorful risk-takers in recent times is a young man named Evel Knievel. Early risk-taking attempts included using a motorcycle to soar over earthbound objects, such as fifty cars parked side by side. In announcing his plans to jump a specially powered motorcycle over the one mile Snake River Canyon in Idaho, he gave as his motive, "I said I would do it, and I intend to keep my word. One of the weaknesses of the U.S. today is that not enough people do what they say they'll do." On September 8, 1974, Evel rode his rocket not across the canyon as proposed, but parachuted into the Snake River when it misfired. A newspaper account reported,

> His (Evel's) barrier, the natural grandeur of the Snake River Canyon, was in itself awesome. His task was formidable—to ride a gerrybuilt 'skycycle' across the yawning chasm and land safely on the other side. Rip-off, it might have been, but the stunt most certainly was not without risk . . . He lost obviously—but it was not the kind of loss that would lead a strategist to state bluntly that losing is nothing.[1]

But of course, behind all of his accomplished and proposed feats of daring is the philosophy, "If there's little risk, there's no reward." Though

---

[1] *Chicago Tribune,* Tuesday, September 10, 1974, Section 3, page 1, Section 3, page 3. Reprinted courtesy of the *Chicago Tribune.*

most of us, particularly adults but some youth also, would not do these risky things . . . and do value safe behavior over the reckless . . . we have some residual feelings of admiration for these daring-do's.

HERO AND COWARD. Another aspect of this essentially physical risk-taking, which we are somewhat ambivalent about in our thinking, is that in conjunction with military combat. The long, drawn-out, generally unpopular war in Indo-China encouraged a great deal of anti-war feeling, which then tended to produce the feeling that military bravery is not very intelligent . . . maybe even stupid. Still, war and combat have been part of our history, inseparable from the position of world prominence the U.S. holds today. The Congressional Medal of Honor is awarded to those few combatants who risk their lives obtrusively, for others or for some worthy objective. Some survive the risk, and others do not. At the other extreme, cowards or traitors are not persons admired by most of us, despite their concern for their own personal safey and survival. So, we value life and we do not presently think highly of war, but we still tend to favor the hero over the coward and to revere and honor the spiritual principle, "Greater love hath no man than this . . . that a man lay down his life for his friends."

MOOD MODIFIERS. Another important, but different area of risk-taking, is that relating to the use of substances that modify mood and behavior. It was reported earlier in this book that health education in schools really was kindled by the temperance movement, whose feelings that young people should know the risks involved in use of alcohol and other narcotizing substances were translated almost universally into state statutes of required teaching-learning. Today, the raison d'être of many health education programs is that youngsters should know the risks involved in use of alcohol, tobacco, and other drug-type substances. For each of several substances, there is a range of attitudes about the risks involved. Statements representative of some of these positions follow.

CIGARETTES

Developing lung cancer, emphysema, or heart disease is nothing that I want to happen to me, and I think smoking does lead to these, so no smoking for me.

I've been smoking for fifteen years, but I've noticed trouble in breathing lately, and I sure don't want to get lung cancer or emphysema . . . and I may be one of the susceptible . . . .

I think smokers are more likely to develop lung cancer, emphysema and heart disease than non-smokers, but I enjoy smoking, so I'm limiting myself to an average of a little less than a pack a day.

I'd like to smoke, but the boy I really like . . . and that I want to like me . . . doesn't like smoking. So having him like me is sure more important than smoking.

I really don't care much about smoking, but most of the girls in this group I really want to be in with do smoke, so I'd sure rather smoke than risk their not accepting me.

Maybe smoking does cause lung cancer, emphysema, and heart disease . . . I like to smoke . . . and I figure if it's my time to go, I'll go, whether I smoke or not . . . I guess I'd say it's a risk worth taking.

BEVERAGE ALCOHOL

When I see and hear about all the trouble that alcohol causes I just resolve over and over again never to drink—or approve of drinking for anyone.

I guess some people can drink and not have any trouble, but I'm not sure how I could handle it, so, for me, non-drinking is the best way to go.

I realize that drunkenness, drunk driving, and alcoholism are real personal and social problems, and I sure don't want to be part of any of these, but I enjoy a drink now and then, so I'll just be careful to always stay moderate.

The group I want to be associated with likes to drink, but my family doesn't approve of drinking, so I drink with the crowd, but am careful not to lose control so that my family would find out that I drink.

Drinking? When people get obnoxious, sloppy, and sick I sure disapprove, but most of the time it makes people happy, friendly, witty, even brave, and I think this is a great way to be.

I like to drink . . . I even like to get drunk. Alcohol may be harmful to some people, but they're probably losers anyway. If there *are* any risks in drinking, they're certainly worth taking.

MARIJUANA

There just isn't enough known about marijuana . . . particularly long-term effects, so I'm not going to take any chances.

From what I hear, marijuana gives a nice, gentle high, but it's still illegal and whatever it might do just isn't worth the possibility of being arrested for possession.

I tried grass once and it made me feel too good. I think I might come to want it too much, so I'm staying away from it.

I like grass, and I smoke it every once in awhile, but my Dad's position in life, which is really important to him, would be so jeopardized if I were busted that I just don't feel comfortable getting stoned.

I'm not sure how I feel about pot, but I really like this group of kids and they like to smoke, so I go along to enjoy what they enjoy and experience what they experience.

I like to smoke and I really enjoy getting stoned. I don't believe there's any harm that can come from pot, and nobody gets convicted for just smoking any more. It's one of nature's nice weeds.

BARBITURATES

You can get hooked worse on barbs than on any other drug. Whatever the high experience might be, it's not worth losing your right to choose.

I realize this Seconal can be really habit-forming, and I'm trying not to become dependent on it, but when I just *can't* go to sleep . . . well, eventually, I just have to take a couple.

It's a beautiful, soft high that lazes right over into delicious sleep. I enjoy it, and I'm certainly not going to worry about any future bogeyman of being hooked.

AMPHETAMINES

I've seen kids strung out on speed . . . and I heard one of them died. They really weren't having any fun . . . just taking more to keep from crashing. I'd like to see anyone try to get me to take any of that stuff.

I don't really like the high experience with benzedrine, but it does get me active. I move around and do things, and I don't feel hungry. I don't like being a drug-taker, but I don't like being fat and lethargic either.

I've done a lot of things, but the greatest of all is to really fly with speed. It's not really addicting, and I can handle any psychological dependency. Anyone who's ever tried it will tell you it's a risk worth running.

HEROIN

I've had opportunities, but I keep thinking that any drug use could eventually lead to heroin, and the thought of ever becoming a junkie and shooting stuff into my arms just sickens me. Nothing is worth that.

I didn't really want to go to H, but these kids I was with just decided that was the big experience we should all have, so what could I do . . . or say.

Sometimes I think I'd like to get off this stuff, but when I feel those pains coming and that dryness in my mouth I get out and hustle some more and nudge my old system off into that beautiful Land of Nod again.

MOOD MODIFYING ANALYZED. So, at one extreme are folks who recognize the dangers and are unwilling to take the risks that are potential and possible. Then there are others who see some personal susceptibility to difficulty. They're not against all use, but they perceive a personal risk not worth running. Next come those who admit some risks but use anyway, but with caution and moderation. Some don't use, or are very moderate, because of the risk of disfavor from someone they wish to please. Conversely, some run whatever risks a substance has because of the desire to be part of a group. Finally, hard core users are those whose perceptions of the using experiences are positive enough to counter any potential or actual danger. They either deny the risk or they see it overshadowed by the using experience. Fortunately or unfortunately, there is far from universal agreement about what is a risk and which risks are worth what real or apparent pleasure.

DRIVING. In one respect, this risk category we've just rambled through leads to another—driving . . . and it also leads to another—sexual relations. Yet these do not seem related to each other. Humm . . . Well, let's first consider the risks in piloting the product of America's foremost industry—the auto. Driving is risky enough so that only experts should drive. Yes, all drivers must pass certain tests to be licensed, but frequently these are inadequate. Some people know that there are more than 50,000 deaths and over two million disabling injuries annually from automobile accidents . . . and everyone knows that there are dangers in driving, but the total miles driven per year continue to rise. In one sense, the risk goes up annually—there are more deaths and injuries each year. In another sense, it goes down—there are fewer per mile driven. You take your choice of perspective.

The automobile undoubtedly would not be so hazardous if drivers could be trained to be careful and courteous and if they did not prepare for their driving as if they were going to be travelling in the Indianapolis 500 mile race. But the automobile is part of an American thing about getting somewhere fast . . . or on time . . . or to two places in the time normally sufficient for one. It is a curious fact that most cars are designed to travel faster than even the highest speed limit, and then officers of the law spend time and energy arresting drivers for exceeding the speed limit. The higher the speed the less control the driver has, except to continue in a straight line. Much driving is very routine, even dull and boring. But driving also is, almost by definition, not completely predictable. A driver may, at any time, be called on to make a decision and execute some control maneuver quickly. During the time the driver is reacting, deciding, turning, braking, or whatever, the car is proceeding as it was, and the faster it was going the farther it goes in the original direction before the maneuver takes it somewhere else. Accidents typically occur during this interim period.

CAR AS POWERFUL ME. The auto can also be perceived, usually unconsciously, as a powerful extension of self. People who feel reckless can express this by kicking a can, swinging from a tree branch, shouting loudly into the wind—or by driving as their reckless feeling dictates. The risks of driving seem to fade away as the exhilaration of speed, power, and omnipotence invades the driver's spirit. Taking a chance in passing a car may seem to be the essence of life. Time can be shortened by speed. Rational behavior can be seduced by speed and power.

Driver education is designed to teach driving in a rational, even defensive way. Yet at this point, there is no indication that it is eliminating those risk-takers from the driving population. For many people, probably more the young but not exclusively, driving can become, in a moment's whim, a delicious game of chance. Most of these are not wild, irresponsible people. But when life seems tedious and boring, as it may for all of us from time to time, the remedy may be a tromp on the accelerator or a screech of tires. And when one driver becomes less predictable, all others around become less also, and the chance for a crash increases. Despite all the present and projected safety measures and precautions, none seem capable of overcoming this need to drive insanely.

SEXUAL EXPRESSION. As pointed out before, there is far from universal agreement about what is a risk and which risks are worth what pleasures. In the past, it was much more evident that sexual relations outside of marriage were risky and much clearer what the dire consequences could be. Much less so today. There is a risk of pregnancy, which for the female certainly has physical consequences, but also potential emotional, social, and spiritual repercussions. The risk of venereal disease is equal for both sexes. But sexual relations, even without pregnancy or venereal disease, can bring unpredictable results. Even within a happy marriage, each time of sexual intimacy has the potential for satisfaction or for frustration. The married couple can usually survive these latter, partly because there are enough of the former. Young Americans probably know as much about the physical aspects of sex as any youth age group ever has, but this knowledge does not seem to reduce the risk factors. One of the important things to realize is that few people can ever really know about sexual relations, because they involve non-predictable personality and emotional interactions with another not completely predictable human being. When the couple is young, immature, unsure of themselves and inexperienced, the risks seem obviously greater.

The risks involved in homosexual relations are the same as for heterosexuals, plus the risk of additional social discrimination . . . even harassment. The general cultural climate is not so completely in support of social ostracism and ridicule as in the past, but neither is it one of open acceptance.

Beyond sex is love in its many forms. The risk involved in loving another person is that the person will not return the love, will not respond in kind. When one genuinely feels love and expresses it, it constitutes an offering of self. Unqualified acceptance with the assurance of mutual love is the supreme goal. To be rejected may be the supreme frustration. Once rejected, can a person risk that again? This seems a far cry from what is more traditionally thought of as health risks—chancing a stomachache or a broken tooth. But the risk of loving may be closer to the heart of people's functioning well, or poorly, than are physical factors.

Two final areas of risk. Learning in school is a risk, as schools are generally set up. The essential risk is that you will not learn what is expected or that you will learn it incorrectly or incompletely. At some point, you will have to demonstrate that you have achieved or have not. To achieve is satisfying. To miss achieving is embarrassing, frustrating, and painful. Those who do learn find it easier to learn more. Those who have not learned find it tempting to stop taking the risks. And this happens not only in schools. A friend of mine has worked for the telephone company for years and is very knowledgeable about virtually all equipment that the company operates. He recently was transferred to supervise six installers, one of whom had a reputation as a lazy troublemaker. My friend discovered that the man had worked for the company for ten years, but had never been trained for this job. Everyone assumed that because of his years of service he should know what he was doing. There had been no easy way for him to learn, so rather than risk the loss of face he took on the role of lazy troublemaker. When my friend started patiently to teach him his job, without any acrimony, he responded beautifully and learned very rapidly.

The last area of risk to mention is choice of life work. The risk is in having to choose before one can really know what it is like. The risk is in choosing something that is satisfying in the younger years,

Risk-Taking   115

but doesn't last. The risk, for a woman, is in deciding on high priority—choosing a career or choosing a man to marry, or both. The contemporary risk is in preparing for some career that will not continue in the future. Who would have predicted that MacGarnosh, receiving his Ph.D. in 1957 and going confidently into the high paying aerospace industry, would be out of a job in 1970, past the point in life of feeling easy and comfortable about starting a new career. Some young people are opting not to join the working culture yet, mostly with some confidence that their ability and/or family position will find them a worthy position when they decide to return to "straight" life. The risk being run is that able peers who seriously complete their education may take the choice jobs, leaving the dropout only undesirable choices.

ANOTHER GAME. In a previous chapter, I commented briefly on the "Game of Adult and Child." Somewhat parallel to this is the "Game of Health Educator and Students." In this game the health educator seems to urge learners to be more cautious (to take fewer risks) than she/he really thinks desirable. (That is, she/he would be a little worried if young learners were as cautious about everything as adult values would suggest). On the other side, the students appear to take (and want to take) more chances than they actually do. I remember a conversation in point with two members of the "hardest drinking fraternity" on a West Coast campus where I taught some years back. I asked, "Do you all drink as heavily as your reputation suggests?" They replied, "No, we have a couple of really hard drinkers . . . the rest of us just ride along on their reputation." Again, the game is largely unconscious, so it can get out of balance fairly easily. The ideal equilibrium is when students are not quite measuring up to health education standards, and yet are following more healthy practices than they would generally admit.

- Health, for most folk, is a matter of balancing risks rather than taking none at all.
- Though the most obvious risks are physical, there are also mental, emotional, social, and spiritual risks.
- Risks may be quite complex—i.e., avoiding a physical risk may mean taking a social and spiritual risk.

WHAT IS HEALTHY? . . . AGAIN. Probably taking some risks, even a few major ones now and again. "Unhealthy" becomes the label when the individual takes too many risks or loses too often. And, of course, there are those fairly rare cases of taking too few risks. Remember, though, healthy is traditionally a conservative value; the assumption underlying this value is that once you have it then you guard it by not taking risks. Being safe is being healthy.

But perhaps this is akin to the librarian who really feels most comfortable when all books are checked back in and are on the shelves. What is a library for? What is health for? To function. To function well, Margi, Charles, Ken, and Barby take some risks, mixed artfully with some precautions. Risk-taking is necessary for healthy functioning. Succeeding where one could fail is the basis for the good, dynamic life. As Margi, Ken, Charles, and Barby succeed, they become better able to succeed in the future. Life in these United States isn't pure survival of the fittest—and shouldn't be—but it is doubtful if any cultural artifacts can negate—or provide a substitute for—the individual who takes a risk (with some caution, perhaps), succeeds, and then more confidently faces the next set of life choices. As a preview to a later chapter: she/he who adapts well increases her/his ability to adapt even better in the future.

Chapter VIII

Getting High

It has been asserted that health education in the schools really got its impetus and start from the temperance movement and its commitment to warn youngsters of the evils of intoxication. Now, more recently, in the early 1970's, many established health education programs have been rejustified on the basis of including education about drugs. Undoubtedly some of the classroom learning experiences genuinely leave youngsters freer (with understanding) to make up their own minds about drug use. However, I would wager that most drug—and alcohol—education communicates directly or more subtly that all experiences of getting and being "high" are undesirable and unhealthy. Since many people—young, middle-aged, and old—behave as though getting an alcoholic high is healthy, it seems appropriate to deal with it here. Remember, too, that one premise and promise of this book is to deal with health-related issues that often are not covered in similar health education literature.

The writings of psychiatrists Andrew Weil [1] and Morris Chafetz [2] tend to support the position identified above. Let's take a closer look at this position.

The health education slogan we must wrestle with first is: *Healthy persons value their rational minds and behave in predictable ways.* There is no way, of course, that this can be faulted . . . except by whispering the tiny question, Always? Then follows the query as to whether the above requires a negative valuing of altered states of consciousness, which are of two basic types:

- more awareness

- more unawareness

Thus, the definition of "getting high" is emerging as "any favorably perceived expansion of the usual, rational use of the mind and normal predictable reaction and behavior." Naturally, it starts from the positive high experiences where something causes an overriding of the routine rational and the normal. Rationality is still present, but it loses its influence in competition with the high. But getting high also includes the stripping away of the rational deterrents to feeling free—those inhibitions the rational mind exerts for our own good. Something

---

[1] Weil, Andrew, "Man's Innate Need: Getting High," *Intellectual Digest,* August, 1972. pp. 69-71.

[2] Chafetz, Morris E., *Liquor: The Servant of Man.* Boston: Little, Brown and Co., 1965. 229 pp.

thus reduces rational controls, one is less aware of them . . . and therefore high.

- Charles has taken a capsule of Y and is experiencing sensations never encountered before. His mind is sharp, but his accustomed way of viewing things just cannot compete with these new sensations. His rational mind chirps, "But wait. . . ." while his altered consciousness thunders, "But wow! What an experience!"

- Fred has taken a capsule of Z, and life is all slowed down. All of the nagging constrictions that usually make him feel normal but slightly uncomfortable have slid back and no longer seem important. It seems as though he has time to feel things, with no clear remembrance about how he should react to them. He is gently floating, high above the restraints of reality . . . but this seems real, too . . . to some usually quiet part of his being.

Each is a high. Each is a favorably perceived departure from the rational mind and from normal reactions. But the sensations are different from one another.

HIGHS COME NATURALLY . . . TO SOME. The most important admission, first of all, is that such high sensations, of both types, come naturally to people—in various kinds of experiences, including the religious. The temperaments of some people are such that they experience these sensations naturally and often, even when others in the same experience situation are not so aware. Others seem naturally able to control their consciousness so that they experience fully or are not unnecessarily inhibited by their own selves. Still others truly cultivate controls over the body and mind, as in meditation. Out of this discipline come experiences that certainly seem beyond the rational, and are constituted highs. And, then, others use chemicals—those that are naturally occurring and/or those concocted and produced in this better-living-through-chemistry era.

THE SPRINTER MUST REST. The frontal lobes of the cerebrum represent that part of the brain that initiates and controls many aspects of functioning, which differentiate human from animal and civilized man from savage. Memory, reasoning, inhibitions, and judgment originate here, and combine in those unique motivations that push humans on to achieve more . . . to be better . . . to be concerned. But, in a Chafetz image,[3] this, part of the brain is akin to the sprinter, and these concentrations of attention, focusing of efforts, evaluating, instituting corrections all are very taxing. Just as the sprinter cannot keep up her/his torrid pace for more than a few hundred yards, the cerebral cortex also must rest periodically from its strivings. Many of our

---

[3] Ibid., pp. 181-182.

reactions truly are returns to the primitive, actually or symbolically—
hiking, swimming, sailing, cooking out, camping. They constitute rest
for the cerebrum. So do some chemical substances, and their effects
often can be felt more quickly.

EXEMPLARY VOYEURISM. Or . . . let's look in on a party or
gathering of young adults, many of whom are not acquainted. Most
of them have learned since childhood that some people you don't know
cannot be trusted. They have learned, as children, that you lock your
bike and your house, that you do not ride with strangers, that some
people can harm you. They have learned that expressing what you think
may not be well received by others. This is all rational, but it is also
uncomfortable.

Some persons are uncomfortable because they feel they are not
smart enough to enter conversations; others may feel edgy because they
have more education than most. Some are naturally shy; others are
nervous about social interacting; some may be downright fearful.

On the other hand, undoubtedly there are some present who
easily "turn on" to people and for whom the gathering in itself is a
natural high. We tend to say, "Bravo for them!" and, "The others
ought to be able to do this, too." Except that it is unlikely that we
all shall ever have this gift of relaxation and heightened pleasure.
And probably all at the gathering need to be freed from some restraints,
some inhibitions. Music may help some . . . finding a compatible con-
versational companion may help some . . . food may help . . . a relaxed
environment may help . . . liquids may help . . . or alcohol, a mood
modifying substance, may help to achieve a high. An analysis as to
why certain males, participants in the California Drinking Practices
Study, did drink to intoxication contained the piquant observation that,
for many of these men, getting drunk is akin to "unbuckling one's
sword." This implies, in the terms being used here, that getting high
with others is an act of trust. The rational mind says, "Be careful . . .
keep your protective sword ready." It is rational, but it is probably
uncomfortable. It is childlike to feel high and it is difficult to trust
people without question. It is healthy for an adult to be childlike—
this does not mean childish.

REALITY is generally defined as our plane of rational consciousness.
It is where we are and what we perceive most of the time. But, says
Chafetz, most of us evidence a "persistent and irradicable desire for
both simulation and narcosis." [4] This implies pushing beyond the
rational consciousness or having its sharp edges buffed away. Reusing
the terms introduced earlier, it implies the desire for "heightened

[4] Ibid., pg. 151.

awareness and heightened unawareness." But each can be sought for good reasons or not-so-good reasons. Getting high can mean flight, escape, and an attempt to lose one's self . . . or it can mean a search, a relief, a relaxation, a fulfillment, a discovery of self. Ethyl alcohol, an active constituent of many familiar drinks and beverages, can induce both feelings—stimulation and narcosis. And it can be used for the whole range of reasons.

RANDOM AND UNPREDICTABLE BEHAVIOR. Human behavior, with the rational consciousness dominating, still is complex and not completely predictable. When people get high on such things as alcohol, their behavior, in general, becomes more random and even less predictable. This becomes worrisome to those who are not high.

- Agnes is high, and is not as critical of herself and of others as usual; this can be good if her normally critical nature alienates people from her . . . and bad if it worsens her critical behavior and alienates even more people.

- Marion is high, and she is more critical of herself and others than she usually is; this is good if it allows her to say something necessarily critical to another that she couldn't say otherwise . . . and bad if it unnecessarily hurts another's feelings.

- When Gary is high, he becomes more affectionate with women and with men. He normally feels affectionate, but he has learned to exhibit the expression of it to fit societal norms. Rationally, he does not want to be considered either homosexual or lecherous, and his sober behavior drips with decorum. However, his behavior, when high, suggests that these inhibitions are not entirely comfortable. Expressing affection and having it returned is, for him, "a beautiful way to function." *

- When Bernie and Jeanne, who are not married to each other, get high at a drinking party, they become affectionate with each other. Their spouses and other friends understand, but it still is worrisome to most of them because of rational projections about what could happen. They are not drunk enough to be oblivious to this so their inclinations to high behavior become a mixed bag—still personally enjoyable, but socially dangerous and potentially punishing. Behavior thus becomes even more unpredictable.

ESCAPE . . . TO . . . AND FROM. Perhaps it is time to revisit that dual concept of escape once again. Getting high may well be an escape,

---

* It is an observable fact that for the majority of American males past puberty there are only two legitimate "scenes" in which physical embracing of other males is condoned. Both of these are "high" occasions. One is in the midst of competitive athletics and the other is when drinking.

but, from the standpoint of health, it can be important. It can be healthy or unhealthy.

TOO MUCH PLEASURE AND RISK. Let us be realistic. The reasons that the general philosophy of this chapter is not good, solid health education dogma are several. Two disparate ones should be sufficient for this treatment.

- The most dominant and compelling ethic in the background of the majority of Americans is a Puritan one, one facet of which is a suspicious feeling about unearned pleasures. This seems far back, and one may be hard-pressed to find a hardcore, thorough-bred, admitted Puritan, but there is still continued evidence of discomfort over one's own pleasures and other people's hedonism. The discomfort may be displayed in overmuch laughter, joking, and fun-making. The point is that the response is other than easy acceptance of high behavior. And though the referent high in this discussion is that from drinking, a great many people would be equally discommoded by someone in the ecstacy of a religious high, marked by uninhibited movements and speaking in tongues.

- Another reason is that most professionals who approach this phenomenon with a minimum of emotion and initial judgment agree with Weil[5] that "the experience comes from the mind, not from the drug." Those who experience agreeable highs are basically experiencing something unusual, but not distinct, from the potentials in their own minds. Likewise, those who experience problems cannot really say, "It wasn't me . . . it was the booze." The wrong people use mood modifiers for wrong reasons—from society's perspective.

NATURAL HIGHS. Perhaps it is time to pursue that partial agreement with the thesis of this chapter voiced earlier—getting high is all right when it comes from a more natural stimulus. This begins with response to nature, particularly the non-human portion of the world. Some people get high, then, from examples such as the following:

- Glimpsing, even standing in, a field of wild flowers or looking closely at and smelling a single perfect rose.

- Seeing the big orange full moon seem to rise into the evening sky (even if its color does come from its being viewed through a blanket of smog).

- Seeing and fondling a litter of soft puppies, just opening their eyes.

- Feeling the strange, haunting beauty of a walk on a really foggy night.

---

[5] Weil, "Getting High." pg. 69.

Some people get high from experiences not as natural as the above, but not as artificial as a quart of beer or a joint of marijuana . . . such as the following:

- Hearing a familiar, beloved symphony performed by a skilled orchestra . . . or the overall sound and feel of a fully amplified rock group.
- Experiencing a gripping drama portrayed by a superb cast on film or live.
- Feeling the tingle of patriotism in some unique setting (as I did once in hearing the Star-Spangled Banner played by the talented string section of a teenage Japanese orchestra, all standing at attention as they played).
- Seeing a child of yours perform in some outstanding fashion.
- Achieving some personal honor, for which you have strived conscientiously.
- Feeling the stimulating glow of exercise and competition in the midst of a volleyball game.
- Feeling the delicious coming on of sleep at the end of a busy day.
- Experiencing the combination of excitement and relaxation in interacting with an attractive member of the opposite sex.

MEDITATION is a practice about which most Americans have some notion. It can be quietly contemplating the meaning of God, of addressing a problem with special thought, or just sitting quietly. Over the past decade, more of us have become aware that it really is a more complex phenomenon. Yet meditation would still be a barely-noticed foreign religious practice if it were not evident that some of our youngsters have turned from drug abuse to meditation. As Weil [6] asserts, "A great many experienced drug takers give up drugs for meditation, but no meditators switch to drugs." So meditation has functional value; we judge drug abuse (even use) to be deleterious, so something that substitutes for it must be good. But meditation is fundamentally another way of getting high, but on a much different principle. Meditation denies the validity of the instant high induced by drugs and upholds the merit of that which follows from controlling and disciplining the mind. Like the undisciplined athlete who, though strong, agile, and fast enough, performs poorly in actual contests, the undisciplined mind blocks itself and prevents its person from truly being aware. Meditation helps develop control of the mind, a side effect of which is greater awareness—a high experience. In meditation, one strives for control and achieves an eventual high.

---

[6] Ibid., pg. 70.

RELIGIOUS EXPERIENCES certainly are acceptable—even commendable—conditions for getting high for many people. Many of the folk who are shocked and disturbed by drug use would applaud the young person who "turns on to Jesus." Some of these experiences are fairly regular and commonplace. For example, feelings of warmth, thrill, and love in singing a congregational hymn, listening to a good choir anthem, hearing an inspiring sermon, participating in a prayer experience, and/or communion or eucharist. Some will come in special camps, retreats, or services (such as candlelight, ecumenical, New Year's Eve), but the highs produced are basically gentle and non-convulsive. However, religious experiences can also be of the most extreme nature—trances, mystic rapture, seeing visions, hearing holy voices, speaking in tongues, interpreting that spoken in tongues, prophesying, and the superb intoxication of the Holy Spirit.

Experiences in the spiritual realm are explainable psychologically. Explainable, but not provable or disprovable, because the core of the experience is a subjective encounter. The only aspects of this that can be quantified are gross symptoms (temperature, blood pressure, perspiration . . .) and reports of subjective experience. That which a person lives through can be called a hallucination because no rational person sees or senses such things. The labeler may not believe such exist (e.g., the throne of God . . . the hand of God in mine), but there is no way, ultimately, to deny the hypothesis that this is a genuine communion with a power greater than all of us. As argued earlier, to the extent that some scientifically oriented folk deny the existence and power of God, they simply are exhibiting a counter dogmatism to an original dogmatism. They can be genuinely skeptical but should soberly admit that if it is unlikely that devout worshippers can experience the world as, say, psychologists do without their at least eight years of undergraduate and graduate education, then it is equally unlikely that they, as psychologists, can experience the supernatural without the giving of self and devotion characteristic of worshippers. According to a long historical parade of people who have reported significant spiritual experiences that elevate them from ordinary life, God provides some pretty memorable highs.

HEALTHY OR UNHEALTHY? Looking at the total phenomenon, how should the profession answer the interrogation, Is getting high healthy or unhealthy? The most honest answer, probably, is quite equivocal: It can be both . . . it can be either. One of the signs of optimum health is that the person functions well in all dimensions of being. If high experiences seem to result in Ricardo functioning better than he does without such experiences, then the high may be a means to a good end. Lolli [7] postulates that maximum functioning results from a right combination of efficiency and inefficiency. Some inefficiency is necessary in order for efficiency to really be efficient. This calls to mind the confusing, irrational, recurring notion that some important things cannot be achieved by direct assault . . . the harder you strive to achieve directly, the less successful you are. When you relax and stop trying, the goal, strangely, comes closer.

MEANS TO A GOOD END. So, the first positive argument is the obvious one for a basically secular, scientific frame of reference with which healthy education is most identified—a means to a good end. Ricardo's body feels and functions better, his mind is fresher, his feelings about people are more positive . . . so he is healthier. But for those who accept a spiritual dimension to well-being, there can be a direct value. The high experience may be a beautiful end in itself. When I walk in the woods and across the rolling pasture on a cold, clear winter night, with crunchy snow underfoot and crackling stars o'erhead, I do not walk so that I shall sleep better, or write better, or lecture better. In fact, it is an alternative to sleeping, writing, or preparing for a class. And it is utterly worthwhile, for me, in and of itself. A high experience may or may not make the experiencer function better in the more accepted, functional dimension. In this context, that would be a secondary valuation. The prime one would be the personal, subjective quality of the experience.

HEALTH-FUNCTIONING. In some cultures, the basic reason for individual good health is simple and clear. A healthy individual can produce more for the state, which makes her/him more valuable; she/he who is unable or unwilling to produce for the state simply has little or no value. In more individualistically oriented cultures, the basic reason for health is much more cloudy and ambiguous. There still is the value on producing, so the healthy person who functions well is valued. But putting value on the individual irrespective of her/his producing implies that health can be desirable, even if an individual is not going to do anything with it. This makes us somewhat uncomfortable, sometimes, and we're tempted to say that a person in good health will behave in ways that are both personally satisfying and socially useful.

STRAIGHTFORWARD OR GAME-PLAYING? What is the best message for health education in relation to experiences of getting high? One general approach is the straightforward one, where the attempt is to be as honest as possible about possible values and potential haz-

---

7 Lolli, Giorgio, "Alcohol and Alcoholism in America Today," in *Alcohol and College Youth.* Proceedings of a conference sponsored by American College Health Association, 1965. pp. 11-12.

ards. The underlying assumption is that the individual is the most able and the most appropriate one to make decisions about what to do and how to balance activity. In another general approach discussed earlier, health education must make any practice sound worse than it is in order to be a useful counterforce to those who make it sound better than it is.

Each approach has some merit. Some learners are going to respond best to the first. Some others truly need the second because they are bombarded too heavily with propaganda for a hedonistic lifestyle. In any classroom, there is likely to be some of each approach.

IT IS AND IT ISN'T. Perhaps you are ready for the fine textured eclectic statement that can encapsulate this chapter. This is the best I can do: the most ideal behavior—the healthiest—is that combination of functional accomplishment and feeling high.

- Bob spades his garden plot in the spring, preparing the soil for planting, and each shovelful of earth and each rolling bead of sweat translates as an exhilarating experience.

- Ann writes a book that is a significant contribution to her field and brings her some royalties, and, in addition, the experience of putting down on paper (for others to read) ideas she has spawned is a continuing genuine high.

- Dave and Enide go to a cocktail party and truly enjoy themselves. Relaxed by the drinks and warmed by the conversations, they talk together afterward in many ways they never have before. The upshot is that he asks her to marry him, she accepts, and being well-matched but unaware of such, they live a subsequent happy life together.

(It might be ideal if substances were not necessary for some people, as they are not for some . . . but in more ways than this, we do not live in an absolutely ideal world.)

Statement continues: less ideal behavior is accomplishing a task well, but having no pleasurable feeling about the process . . . .

- Steve is a good mechanic and his customers trust his judgment and compliment his work, but for him it's just a job.

. . . or having a high experience that accomplishes nothing tangible, but seems to harm no one either. . . .

- Henrietta leaves work on Friday, drives to the mountains, climbs a difficult peak, savors the experience, comes home, and goes back to work on Monday.

Statement concludes: the least desirable behavior is when the attempted high does not produce the desired feeling, and results in harm to the individual and others.

- Jake is talked into trying cocaine. Not only doesn't he enjoy the experience, but he is arrested for possession of an illegal narcotic drug. He loses his job, his wife and children are put in need, his parents are ashamed. . . .

BALANCE AND APPRECIATE. As life goes on, each of us lives as an individual, but also relates to others. One expected health education imperative is for each of us to balance the possible values and potential dangers of highs and help those we care about to do the same. The unexpected imperative is the additional one of appreciating our own positive, constructive high experiences, and those of others, even if these be different from our own.

Chapter IX

Health
and Health Education
in Ecological Perspective

It began in the early 1960's. The word ecology that we vaguely remembered from general education as describing a branch of biology began to appear in health education literature. But more as a word than as an important, revolutionary concept. In 1964, Professor Howard Hoyman [1] of the University of Illinois presented the field with a paper entitled "An Ecologic View of Health and Health Education," in which he said . . . and asked:

> A man's level of health and disease, his rate of aging, and his length of life are all *dynamic ecologic resultants* . . . more and more, the basic theory and practice of public health is being recognized as *ecologic*. Where do we go from here?

The answer did not come back in any discernible roar of interest.

In 1969, Dr. John Hanlon [2] called his Presidential Address to the American Public Health Association, "An Ecologic View of Public Health." He encouraged dealing with the "complexity of the relationship of *total* man to this *total* environment." This is true . . . and good . . . but it still seemed to stop short of an ecologic view. Hanlon went on to say, however:

> . . . it is our conceptual approach to the man-environment relationship and the quality of it that can lend perspective to what is wrong, how it went wrong, and what ought to be done to right it . . . it is our concepts that in the final analysis shape our public health efforts.

A DISTURBING CONCEPT. Translated, this suggests that health education, as practiced in classrooms, community groups, homes, and through the various media, will not become more influenced by ecology until the concept of ecology is made more understandable.

The professionals who have written histories of the United States up until this past decade were not, for the most part, deliberately falsifying historical analysis. The concept simply was generally accepted

---

[1] Hoyman, Howard S., "An Ecologic View of Health and Health Education," *The Journal of School Health.* 35: 110, 114, No. 3, March 1965. © 1965, American School Health Association, Kent, Ohio 44240.

[2] Hanlon, John H., "An Ecologic View of Public Health," *American Journal of Public Health,* 59: 4-5, January 1969.

that the history of the U.S.A. was fundamentally a history of white people, carving a dynamic nation out of a virgin and partly hostile continent. The newer, developing concept is that Indians were the original native Americans and have a history intertwined with the whites. Black and Chicanos too are Americans who were part of the history. A good deal of the carving of the continent was reckless and wasteful rather than heroic. This blooming concept means that history will have to be rewritten; the old and the familiar can no longer be defended. The perspective must be broadened. Ecological perspective carries a like potential for forcing the rethinking of premises for health education. It may not be pleasant. But it is no longer defensible to pretend that it does not exist.

In his original paper (and in a subsequent one), Hoyman [3] offered the model of a vertical continuum of health for any population, and, ultimately, for any individual. At the top he placed "optimum health—a theoretical level at which an individual's living approaches his full desirable potentialities." At the bottom was "death—extending from so-called 'clinical death' to cessation of life (zero health)." Between these poles were four other levels: critical illness, major illness, minor illness, and wellness.

A HOW BEST CONTINUUM. To begin the development of the concept of ecological perspective, let us consider another continuum. This one contains two poles as divergent interpretations of how best to remain high on Hoyman's vertical continuum—i.e., toward health and away from death. The raison d'être of health education is the opportunity to help individuals learn how to achieve and maintain wellness and health. The question of how best to achieve this favored dynamic state of being seems to be the most relevant concept to the practice of the profession.

THE ECOLOGICAL POLE. One extreme of this proposed continuum is the ecological, where people are seen as a form of life, somewhat unique, but not necessarily better than other forms of life . . . such as camels, cockatoos, crayfish, and Coxsackie viri. The key to health in this extreme view is the capacity for adaptation to the world and all other forms of life.

Ecological perspective affirms that all forms of life have in common the continuous function of food-gathering, ingestion, digestion, absorption, assimilation, and utilization. Every form of life either is or is part of the food supply for another form or forms. Life ultimately,

---

[3] Hoyman, Howard S., "Our Modern Concept of Health," *Journal of School Health,* 32: 254, September 1962.

then, is forged out of dead bodies. Death is a natural and inevitable consequence of having come into being. Death can be a means of renewed and rejuvenated life for others.

The basic principle of ecology is equilibrium. Each individual survives best when it establishes an equilibrium with its ecosystem. Life for any species is maintained best if that species is in equilibrium with other species. The *Tao of Lao-Tzu* describes the benefits of the passive aspect of human adaptation, generally undervalued in Western culture, thusly:

> Those who flow as life flows
> Feel no wear, feel no tear
> Need no mending, no repair.[4]

Ecology portrays a coming to equilibrium, then, as the dominant force in nature. But this is eternally necessary because in the dynamics of relationships among life forms, each form has motivations to be predominant—to survive in greater numbers, at the expense of other life forms. Health adaptation involves an artistic balance (somewhat unique for each individual) between passive acceptance of things as they happen and active effort to change relationships or the environment for mutual benefit. Human beings certainly exhibit this tendency to dominate as strongly as any species . . . and educated Western people, with their scientific medicine, technology, and myriad institutions, epitomize this championing of one form of life.

THE MEDICAL-TECHNOLOGICAL-INSTITUTIONAL POLE. Thus, the more people seek to dominate nature and control other forms of life (rather than establishing equilibrium with them), the more they move toward the extreme antithesis of an ecological view—a view that says that the world **must** be adapted to humans for their comfortable survival. The human being has a brain that can reason, remember, judge, and predict what will happen, given certain circumstances She/he also has hands with opposable thumbs, making the development of technology possible. As a mode of ecological survival, people developed scientific medicine, a growing, reproducing technology, and a variety of institutions designed to make life easier, more efficient, and less painful for human individuals. But their use of these often is anti-ecological.

THE POLES OF A CONTINUUM. Let us look at the poles of this continuum, contrasting the extreme views of what constitutes the best health for the human being—and the human race.

---

[4] Dubos, Rene, *Mirage of Health*. Garden City: Doubleday & Co., Anchor Books, 1961. pg. 210.

ECOLOGICAL			MEDICAL-TECHNOLOGICAL-INSTITUTIONAL	
.	.	.	.	.
1	2	3	4	5

Ecological Pole

Medical-Technological-Institutional Pole

a. Focus is long-range — healthy species result when the strong survive by natural selection; a healthy species is made up of healthy individuals

a. Focus is short-range—on individuals; weak must be made strong; healthy individuals constitute a healthy species

b. Key to health is establishing equilibrium with the environment in a natural fashion

b. Keys to health are improving the individual's internal environment so he/she overcomes threats more easily, and adjusting the environment so it is minimally threatening to individuals

c. Individuals valued as a part of the species according to inherent capacity to adapt to total environment—physical, mental, emotional, and social

c. Each individual is valued, irrespective of weaknesses; the weak have a basic right to be made relatively stronger

d. Some individuals will lose out; this is inevitable and ultimately good for the health of future generations

d. No individual should lose out—no one should be sick or inadequate; human beings must increase their efforts to build up the losers, repair damages, and work for the survival of all

IN SHORT: Individual must adapt to the total environment with her/his own resources

IN SHORT: Individuals must be helped to adapt to the environment — and it must be manipulated in favor of all peoples' survival

Important clarifying announcement: the poles of a continuum are typically uninhabitable. They simply set the stark standard that is finally valued over its stark opposite. Using the numbering system above, a person whose values would put him/her at 2.8 would be virtually indistinguishable from a person at 3.2. However, a 2.5 would see life somewhat differently than a 3.5, and a 2.0 and a 4.0 would disagree on many major assumptions about desirable and undesirable.

What, then, is ecological perspective? It is urging people to look at situations and health-related issues in terms of the relationships among all forms of life in the ecosystem. And, in addition, to anticipate how the environment and other life forms may react and respond to the human's myriad attempts to dominate. Health education has assumed that the human being is a unique, special creature, whose survival and well-being are achieved both by modifying her/his environment and living in harmony with it. Medical sciences and the practice of modern medicine often attempt to prolong the life of one individual who would die without such intervention, which seems anti-ecological. Yet, remember that a more basic premise, already stated, is that each species (and individuals and groups within that species) may not be content with equilibrium and will attempt to adapt in ways that dominate other elements of the ecosystem and make for more and better survival than would be its normal lot. Humans do this . . . and some are quite good at it. Any movement away from equilibrium activates forces to restore equilibrium.

Another way of conceptualizing this is that there are ecological relationships involving Individual Human, Other Living Things (including other humans), Physical Environment, and Culture. In diagrammatic form, it appears thusly (with the non-straight lines symbolizing a dynamic, not entirely predictable, set of interactive relationships):

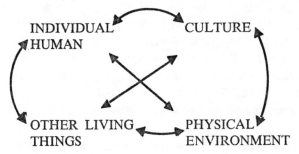

The individual, always the ultimate focus for health in a society, affects other living things and, in turn, is affected by them. She/he manipulates the environment, and the environment also affects the way she/he functions. She/he is molded in certain ways by her/his culture, but by some individual acts she/he may help to change that culture. All of this goes on in more ways than can be charted . . . perhaps even imagined. The individual is faced with threats from other living things (viruses, teachers, peers), from the physical environment (cold, noise, heat, earthquake, smog, speeding automobile), and from the culture (punishing certain behaviors, encouraging other hazardous behaviors). But she/he also may have help in meeting these threats from other living things (parents, teachers, friends, health educators, doctors), from the environment, and from the culture. Often the critical factor in adapting, or reestablishing equilibrium, is the total personal resources of the individual to meet the threat, whatever it may be.

And thus, we are back to the fundamental difference in emphasis between the two sides of the continuum developed earlier. On the left, the ecological, the emphasis is on developing the various capacities to

adapt, inherent in the individual. On the right, the M-T-I, the emphasis
is on providing effective means to deal with threats so that personal
adaptation is unnecessary. A couple of contrasting examples:

- Jack decides he is going to swim across the Mississippi River
during the spring flood state. Without telling anyone, he plunges
in from Missouri and heads for Illinois. His survival, and the
accomplishment of his goal, are now dependent on his strength,
endurance, developed swimming ability, capacity to dodge floating
objects, capacity to endure the cold water, capacity to keep calm,
rest when necessary, and also to keep his bearings so that he is
always moving in the right direction. When he makes it, he has
done it on his own. If he does not, it represents an instance of the
physical environment posing too much of a threat.

- George suffers from a neurological dysfunction that requires that
his breathing be done by an iron lung. He lives and accomplishes
certain goals, but his survival is entirely dependent on forces
beyond his personal control. Science and technology are responsible for the lung; professionals and technicians see that it operates
as it should. Power plants generate electricity that comes by an
intricate route to the machine. As long as these complex interactions continue, George lives. A breakdown in any part may mean
his life, because he has a very minimal capacity to adapt on his
own.

Another example: Robert makes a trip to San Francisco. He flies
from St. Louis on a 727, where his safety and progress are almost
entirely dependent on technology and other people manipulating that
technology, making judgments, etc. After landing, he drives from the
airport to the city, and now his safety and progress are partly dependent
on technology and others, but partly on himself also. He parks several
blocks from the hotel and walks the remainder of the way. His safety
and progress are still dependent to some extent on cultural controls on
traffic, law enforcement, etc., but to a large extent now on his own
personal judgments and adaptations to danger. Arrival at his destina-
tion is, like many of the experiences of modern life, a combination of
personal adaptations and dependence on technology, institutions and
responsible others.

SOME ECOLOGIC SLOGANS. This time during the later 1960's and
1970's in which we have been developing the concept of ecology has
produced some slogans that put truth in intriguing little packets. My
favorite has been:

You can't just do one thing.

This implies that a projected action, though it may solve a problem well, will also have some other effects that at least should be anticipated. Other ways of saying this are:

Everything is connected to everything else.
Everything has to go somewhere.
Nature knows best.
There is no such thing as a free lunch.[5]

Some of the ways that these apply are fascinating, provocative, and even frightening. For example:

- One basic driving premise of our society has been, and continues to be, that use of muscle power, animal or human, is to be supplanted by electrical or mechanical power. The good life thus is translated as doing as little as possible with muscle power and as much as possible with generated power. This is ironic at a time when the calorie intake in foods is as high as in any large culture in the world, with resulting obesity as an expanding health problem. We have experienced rather phenomenal success with this, and have advertised the fact that we produce ample food for our population and have some surpluses for the hungry elsewhere with the least use of manpower in history. However . . .

There is no such thing as a free lunch.

Our production of ample and surplus food has become inextricably linked to use of fossil fuel and electric power. The manufacture of farm machinery, of fertilizer, of pesticides, herbicides, and fungicides, the planting, spraying, reaping, storing, transporting, and processing of various food products require few muscles and many, many kilowatts of energy and gallons of fuel. We have made the transition . . . we have freed man from labor . . . and we have developed a vital system absolutely dependent on fuel of which we have a decreasing supply. The lunch is advertised as a bargain, but before we get out, the cover charge may seem excessive.

On to the next example:

- Population control is equal to pollution reduction as a symbol of better ecological relationships. But population control is all focused in diminishing births, with tacit approval of longer life spans for present adults. The replacement of children with older people in the population will be increasingly costly in energy and pollution.

Everything is connected to everything else.

Though it is risky and premature now, in the future it is possible that the phrase "Nature knows best" could apply.

---

[5] Commoner, Barry, *The Closing Circle*. New York: Alfred A. Knopf, 1972. pp. 33-48.

IS THIS US? At this point, it is difficult to know what is a crisis and what is not. The following analogue may help indicate why.

> A man has a pond. On this pond is a water lily that is multiplying geometrically or exponentially in such a way that in thirty days it will cover the pond and eliminate all other forms of life. He decides not to take any action until the pond is half covered. Following this formula he begins action on the twenty-ninth day and has only one day to avert the disaster.

The energy crisis in which we must decide on priorities for power—food production, sophisticated medical care, heating, cooling, transportation, defense, entertainment . . . may be close. It is difficult to know. It is easy to condemn electric knives, toothbrushes, and can openers, but these are insignificant. What will tend to be critical are such things as convenient but partially filled jet aircraft, unused defense equipment, a car for every driver, and comfortable air conditioning all summer. These could be hard decisions.

HARD REALITIES. An ecological perspective for health education might seem timely, but some probing of its implications presents us with several hard realities, which we must consider and deal with. Some of these are:

1. *Short-range vs. Long-range View.* Health opts for some long-range goals, but also seems, increasingly, to prefer short-term accomplishments. An ecological health message is virtually always long-range, related to as many of the total consequences as are discernible. A conflict in Los Angeles County in the early 1970's involved one physician who advocated preventing venereal disease by using prophylactic tetracycline—because cases actually were significantly less in an experimental trial—in disagreement with his superior who foresaw the consequences of organisms mutating and adapting to the drug so that they could be ultimately more destructive than at present. An obvious case of short- vs. long-range thinking.

   A short-range view of population pressures says, "Heave a sigh of relief that we Americans are now close to zero population growth, which means that more and more people in the future can have a better and better life." A long-range view counters, "Limiting the population certainly means that things are not as bad as they could be. However, the raw materials for the life support of the people of the world are now seen as finite (certainly not unlimited). Americans, with about 5% of the world's population (and diminishing), use over one third of the natural resources—and would use more if the standard of living went up as a result of a stabilized population."

A short-range view of quality protein in the diet says: Animal protein is the highest quality, and the American standard of living will soon make it possible for everyone to eat some meat weekly and for a larger and larger portion of the population to afford as much as they wish. A long-range view retorts: The American eating of meat must decrease to come closer to the diet possibilities of most of their fellow human beings. Americans consume nearly a ton of grain a year per capita, about five times as much as a citizen of India. However, about 90 percent of the American's ton is what has been converted to meat. In the presence of virtually no available meat for many of the world's people, American affluence is accentuated by a dogfood commercial of the early 1970's in which the product is "all meat," and the closing question is, "Doesn't your dog deserve all meat?" Put in population terms, if all the world ate as Asians do there would be enough food at present production levels for five billion people (nearly twice the present population). At American standards there would be enough for less than than one billion (about one third of the present population).

However, a short-range view of sources of energy suggests we shall exhaust major supplies of fossil fuels in the foreseeable future and be unable to sustain present industrialization. A long-range view counters that nuclear energy from fission or fusion and energy from movement of the oceans and the sun will be available. People will have virtually unlimited energy without waste and with moderate cost. There is such a thing as a "free lunch."

2. *Life is Not Problems to Solve.* Scientific thinking encourages a problem-solving approach to life, but problem-solving requires an initial delimiting process so that the problem can be clearly defined and a solution proposed and tested. Delimiting shortens the range, and, hence, the problem no longer represents the reality of life, because of many of the relationships emanating from it are ignored.

Ecological thinking suggests that most health-related issues ARE NOT So Much Problems to Solve as RELATIONSHIPS TO UNDERSTAND—some of which MIGHT BE CHANGED and others simply LIVED WITH.

Modern marital difficulty, for instance, is not a problem to solve, but a result of allowing more individual freedom, which can be had only at the expense of stability. Alcoholism is not a simple problem to solve, but a result of the interaction of some troubled, susceptible personalities in a rather competitive culture with a substance used responsibly and happily by most of their fellow citizens. The latest attempts at therapy for this condition seem to be less oriented to solving the problem and more concerned with helping the alcoholic function more satisfactorily, even if she/he continues to drink.

The complexity of relationships that go beyond the problem-solving model include those instances where the solution to a problem becomes the root of another. In the early 1900's, a leading Philadelphian is reported to have hailed the advent of the motor car because it would help do away with drunken horseback riders and wild horses. And it virtually did! Another example . . . required immunization of all children entering school was a solution to the problem of smallpox, but it created one of deaths from the immunization. That solution is now being reconsidered. And another . . . in the social realm, the obvious solution to the problem of people without adequate housing (i.e., build more houses) would virtually denude the forests still left in this country.

But the complexity includes other instances where one problem becomes the solution to another. Though we do not like to think in these terms, premature death of some young people, as the result of, say, an auto accident, provides a source of kidneys to transplant to those in such need. And . . . a shortage of meat in this culture could reduce consumption, help reduce arteriosclerosis, and contribute to longer life.

Life, then, is not a string of problems, but a network of relationships. An ecological perspective does not imply, as the problem approach seems to, that life is the predicament that precedes death.

3. *A Different View of Death.* Our present health environment tends to view death always as the ultimate enemy, with the companion presumption that virtually all individuals should live longer than they do. Ecological thinking, on the other hand, sees death as a natural consequence of coming into being and a necessary one for the healthy continuation of a species, as well as those for whom that species is a food supply. Further, individuals of a species are not created equal and do not adapt equally to the threats in the ecosystem. As long as people strive, with their medicine, technology, and institutions, to prolong the life of all individuals, it will be at the expense of the rest of the environment. And this will continue as long as health education, in its various forms, displays a basic attitude of ill-will toward death.

BASIC ASSUMPTIONS. Now, let's be practical. Health education is going to be done by a range of professionals and other folk. This means that a range in their positions, their personal beliefs and general outlook on life would place them on the continuum on pages 129-130. It is clear, from working with the continuum model personally and having several classes of university students (including some in teacher education) deal with it, that any individual might be approximately 2.0 in considering one issue (such as the use of auto seat belts) but be perhaps 4.5 in considering another issue (such as taking a daily vitamin pill). But, theoretically, all of an individual's many judgments would average out to some medium that would represent a central-tendency view of life.

A second hypothesis would be that within any health education class group there will be represented a fairly wide range of basic positions—as well as positions on any possible issue worthy of educational consideration. I tested this in a very preliminary way with a class of thirty-five junior level students in a professional health education course. After dealing with this concept in a variety of ways for several sessions, the class members were asked to represent their personal position on the scale and describe, in words, what that meant. For this class, the range was 1.4 to 4.7, with a mean of 3.1. This represents a fairly wide span of basic differences in frame of reference for a class group. According to modern communication theory, an individual's frames of reference include the nature of what she/he perceives—and therefore is able to learn. The farther any learner is from the communicator in basic assumptions, the less likely that predictable learning will take place.

But what does this basic assumption notion really mean? Consider some specific issues. Assuming that the polar positions, representing the extremes as to what will be necessary for best health, can be encapsulated thusly:

	*		*		*	
1	2	3	4	5

Individual must adapt to the total environment	Individual must be helped to adjust to the environment—and it should be manipulated in favor of everyone's survival

Let us consider smoking cigarettes as a specific example issue.

What would Charlie's position of 1.5 (as shown by the left asterisk) represent?

Well, Charles believes that: Smoking is a risk to health and life to which some individuals can adapt and some cannot. Some smokers will succumb to illnesses provoked by smoking early in their smoking careers; others will finally be affected by smoking, but it will take much longer. Still others will adapt to smoking and never seem to be adversely affected by it. With other life dangers reduced, smoking presents a risk, but one that helps keep the population in check.

Another issue: Use of Alcohol Beverages

Wendy's position = 3.0 (the middle asterisk)

Wendy believes: Some individuals will adapt to the effects of alcohol, will control their use, and have few, if any, problems with it. It is inevitable that others will lose some amount of control and will be harmed by the effects. The society needs education about possible effects so that some inadequacies can be recognized early and further loss of control prevented. Of those who lose out some will recover and be rehabilitated. The society needs treatment and rehabilitation services so that some may recover. The cost of recovery for all, however, will be too high.

A third issue could be Automobile Accidents. What would Aaron's 4.5 (the far asterisk) represent?

Aaron believes: With much improved engineering, education, and law enforcement, there should be no accidents. With more and better education for drivers, safer cars, better highways, and a well-functioning enforcement system that denies driving privileges to those likely to have accidents, all accident conditions can be diminished almost to zero.

The interested reader is encouraged to translate each of the positions (or immediate ones) into an interpretation of each of those three issues—and of the gaggle of other issues legitimately part of the health education subject matter.

SOME QUESTIONS. Are those in the health education profession at all homogeneous in relation to a central tendency on this scale? Are most clearly between 3 and 5, definitely favoring the Medical-Technological-Institutional pole? How would an Ecologically-oriented health educator be different from a Medically-Technologically-Institutionally-oriented one? Is it important to know where one stands? What are the implications of each tendency for the health of individuals—and of humans as continuing beings?

A TENTATIVE ANSWER TO THE LAST QUESTION ABOVE MIGHT BE: Medical-Technological-Institutional tendency: The highest value is the survival of all human beings. Weak individuals must be made strong, so services of all kinds (medical, surgical, nutritional, counselling, rehabilitation, etc.) must be increased to assure more than survival—i.e., a high quality of individual human health. The environment must be manipulated and constantly improved, which means made more compatible to people's needs and less hazardous for them. Individuals must live with care and caution—for themselves and for others. The level of risk-taking must be quite low.

Problems inherent in this extreme are (1) an ever increasing population with possible increasing weaknesses; a population of individuals increasingly less able to adapt to unpredicted hazards as they arise, (2) manipulation of the environment for present, individual needs may bring on greater problems for the next generation.

Ecological tendency: The highest value is survival of the fittest, meaning those most able to adapt creatively to the world as it is. The individual must adapt as much as possible without outside assistance. Risk-taking is important as a constant exercise in adaptation and survival—important to the continuing strength of the species.

Problems obvious in this extreme are (1) there will always be losers or those who cannot adapt; (2) there has to be an unwillingness to aid people now when that aid could have foreseen negative consequences for the future.

A THREE-DIMENSIONAL LOOK AT FITNESS. Survival for the majority of *homo sapiens* alive in the world today is still fundamentally physical or biological. The fit are those who survive inadequate diets, multiple infestations of microorganisms, natural threats of storm and drought, and perhaps, the ravages of wars of which they are but passive observers. For Western men and women, including the majority of Americans, the stresses are not so much physical as they are emotional, mental, and social. The individual whose intelligence is not sufficient for a decent grasp of modern life, the persons whose emotions (anxiety, tension, fear, anger, envy, greed) impede adequate functioning, and the individual whose relations with others afford no satisfaction or even are a source of persistent pain—these are the losers of modern life. They survive, biologically, but they basically are unfit for the world in which they survive.

THE FREEDOM ELEMENT. Perhaps many health education professionals are a bit piqued by this time, certain of the rightness of a strong inclination toward the medical-technological-institutional pole, but the ecological principle prevails that no advantage beyond equilibrium comes without its price. The survival of all demands limitation of individual freedom. Risk-taking must be controlled—for the good of all. The ecological pole offers the freedom to adapt and survive and the freedom to fail. When there is no failure, there can be only comparable success. Dubos[6] contends that:

> . . . too often the goal of planners is a universal gray state of health . . . this kind of health will not rule out and may even generate other forms of illness, the boredom which is the penalty of a formula of life when nothing is left unseen.

HUMAN ECOLOGY. I am fully aware that this is a reasonably well accepted term now, but I am still not completely convinced that there is not something anachronistic about it. Hanlon[7] states:

> . . . human ecology places man at the center of concern. It views him as the ecological dominant and recognizes that, while he is a biological organism, his position in the scheme of things is greatly accentuated by the uniqueness of his cerebral capacities, by the culture and society of his fashioning, as well as by the entirety of his surroundings which . . . he has profoundly altered.

It is basically anti-ecological for any species to dominate at the expense of other life forms. I can only conclude, then, that human ecology represents something like a 3.0 position on the proposed scale—a consideration for ecological consequences but a conviction that people must dominate.

ADAPTATION: THE KEY HEALTH BEHAVIOR. All of this leads back again to the exposition of the key to good health (which is the quality of total human functioning)—adaptation. Those who are healthy are those who adapt best . . . to whatever conditions that confront them. Adaptation will range from the very active, vigorous attempts to change some aspects of things (i.e., culture, physical environment, and other living things) to the very passive acceptance of things as they are. But it is an ecological fact that what people use to help them adapt may become threats to their future functioning. A recent newspaper account described a farmer whose prosperity had been greatly enhanced by the tractor, models of which he had operated for twenty-five years. Nevertheless, he was killed when his latest model overturned and crushed him. A young couple glories in the birth of their first child. At the same time, a middle-aged couple agonizes as their first child, now a teenager, lies silent and uncommunicative, the result of a psychotic break induced by repeated use of some identified drug substance.

AGAIN. To reiterate, those means a person uses to adapt to the needs of life may, immediately or eventually, become threats to which she/he must then adapt. Penicillin, a Volkswagen bus, a six pack of Budweiser, marriage, a letter from a good friend . . . each and all can be means of

---

[6] Dubos, *Mirage of Health,* pg. 210. By permission of Harper & Row.
[7] Hanlon, "An Ecologic View of Public Health." pg. 9.

adapting, but can also become a threatening aspect of a person's environment. For the individual's total environment has dimensions that are physical, mental, social and spiritual.

- The basic principle of ecology is equilibrium.

- Healthy ADAPTATION involves the individual achieving a balance between passive acceptance of things as they are and active effort to change things.

- Ecological perspective means anticipating how the environment and other life forms are likely to respond to people's many attempts to modify nature.

- Individuals learn to adapt (or cope) by adapting to real situations, where there is some risk of failure. To eliminate the possibility of failure is to take away the need to adapt.

- The individual who does not need to adapt may lose the capacity to do so . . . should it ever be necessary.

LISTEN TO THE EXPERTS. Health educators new to the current arena of ecological exposition may incline toward listening to an expert. But it is important to realize the differences that separate the better known ecologists. Paul Ehrlich[8] and John Holdren[9] currently see our drives for influence and the size of our population as the twin causes for the worsening ecological situation. For them, population control is the major need of the present—as the means of curbing the rate of natural resource use. Barry Commoner[10] and Buckminster Fuller[11] seem presently little concerned with limiting population, but are much alarmed by our faulty and unwise use of technology. Rene Dubos,[12] the despairing optimist, feels that people's capacity to adapt may be so great that they will adapt to increasingly intolerable changes—and create an equally intolerable existence.

Peter Farb[13] offers another intriguing perspective:

Man is the only creature that seemingly stands aloof from the interactions of living things, since he is able to make a home for himself almost anywhere in the world. But impressive as his accomplishments are, man in reality has never left his ecological

---

[8] Ehrlich, Paul R., *The Population Bomb.* New York: Ballantine Books, 1968. pp. 17-35, 66, 67.

[9] Ehrlich, Paul R. and Holdren, John P., "Hidden Effects of Overpopulation," *Saturday Review.* pg. 52, August 1, 1970.

[10] *Commoner, The Closing Circle.* pp. 139, 231.

[11] Fuller, R. Buckminster, *Earth, Inc.* Garden City: Anchor Press/Doubleday, 1973. pp. 67, 75-77, 175-208.

[12] Dubos, Rene, *Man Adapting.* New Haven: Yale University Press, 1965. pp. 274-279.

[13] From *Ecology* by Peter Farb and the Editors of TIME-LIFE Books, © 1963, 1970 Time Inc. pp. 10, 165.

home . . . man belongs *to* nature and cannot long remain separate from various biological laws without an eventual day of reckoning—that he must develop what the American conservationist Aldo Leopold called an ecological conscience.

Perhaps man is most human when he is following his well-developed conscience and thinking of others rather than himself —in the future as well as in the present.

But Paul Ehrlich [14] suggests that any change in our present course is not a simple intellectual one. Rather

Our entire system of orienting to nature must undergo a revolution. And that revolution is going to be extremely difficult to pull off, since the attitudes of Western culture toward nature are deeply rooted in Judeo-Christian tradition. Unlike people in many other cultures, we see man's basic role as that of dominating nature, rather than as living in harmony with it. . . . Both science and technology can clearly be seen to have their historical roots in natural theology and the Christian dogma of man's rightful mastery over nature.

Ehrlich feels that historian Lynn White [15] makes the dilemma quite clear:

Both our present science and our present technology are so tinctured with orthodox Christian arrogance toward nature that no solution to our ecologic crisis can be expected from them alone. Since the roots of our trouble are so largely religious, the remedy must also be essentially religious, whether we call it that or not.

WHERE ARE WE NOW? We live in a culture with medicine, technology, and institutions that have been developed as helpful means of adaptation. Yet these often are utilized to dominate other life forms and the environment, upsetting the ecological balance. At the same time, this culture is competitive, and the strong function better. One of the challenges of health education in this decade is to help young learners to see where we are as a culture and where various subcultures are. The subsequent challenge is to help them understand positions other than their own, appreciate the range of possible behaviors in any situation, and have some feel for the values that motivate different individuals to different life-styles. Above all, the functional understanding of relationships of all kinds may be fundamental content and process that will keep health going throughout.

---

[14] Ehrlich, *The Population Bomb.* pp. 170-171. From *The Population Bomb,* revised edition, © 1968, 1971 by Paul R. Ehrlich. Reprinted by permission of Ballantine Books, a division of Random House, Inc.

[15] White, Lynn, "The Historical Roots of Our Ecologic Crisis," *Science,* 155: 1206-1207, March 10, 1967.

Chapter X

Some March
to
Different Drums

Chapter I, in its exposition on the nature of this book, offered the somewhat oblique thought that ". . . there are many more differences among U.S. folk than health education has assumed in the past. Effectiveness may increase with the realization and serious consideration of individual and group differences." The pages in this chapter will try to explicate this vital idea.

It really is a matter of valuing. Values underlie an individual's attitudes and motives, which combine to predispose her/him to act in certain reasonably predictable ways. Each person shares certain values with others, yet rare would be the occurrence of even two people with completely identical values . . . and even rarer an individual with an absolutely unique value shared with no other human. Sociologists, who study various groups of people in a culture, devised the concept of social class, asserting that certain social and economic values and behaviors would be shared by segments of the population, which would cut across other lines—like race, religion, sex, geographic origin.

Today, a new understanding of society has revealed that the old social class stereotypes do not hold, making it difficult to generalize. For example, there may be as many differences among individuals labeled "middle class" as there are similarities.

Professional health educators are not all alike. As groups within the culture develop and exhibit more diversity from one another, the need for even greater health education variation may increase. A general observation would be that health educators vary across a continuum between

Almost Any	Particular
Behavior as	Specified
Long as It	Behaviors and
Helps a	Non-Behaviors
Person Function	for Health

.   .   .   .

I have seen no evidence presented or guesses hazarded as to where a central tendency for present practitioners would be. Health textbooks would seem to be definitely toward the right side—toward fairly specific behaviors. But this is all very abstract and theoretical. How does it all translate to what people feel and do?

WHAT AND HOW TO EAT should be a good first example. The prevailing values for health education are most likely to be: (1) daily meals should provide a balance of the essential nutrients, provided by a balance of foods from the Four Food Groups: (2) protein is essential, and meat, being the best source of high quality protein (all the amino acids needed) should be eaten; and (3) eating in patterns that produce obesity (weight ten percent or more over recommended poundage) should be avoided. These dominant values reflect the specific behaviors indicated on the right side of the continuum.

How could a health educator respond to the following variations—reflecting somewhat different values represented by the left side of the continuum?

Variant	Possible Response
"We have very little money to spend on food. . . . By the time we buy those things we always have eaten and like to eat, there's usually not enough money for foods that would make a better balance."	"Let's explore all the foods you've always eaten and like and see what possible new combinations could achieve a better balance. How about an initial goal of one balanced meal a week and working toward one a day. . . ?"
"I'm fat and I know it, but I see no point in punishing myself by dieting. I like to eat, and I'm going to eat what I like for as long as I live."	"The health risks from obesity are less when you don't smoke and do exercise. There are healthier ways to be fat . . . and if you keep your mental outlook positive and happy, that, too, can be in your favor."
"People have no right to take the lives of animals for their own selfish purposes. Eating meat is barbarian. Being a strict vegetarian like I am keeps your mind clear and open to vibrations that meat eaters just can't experience."	"I'd bet your best vibrations would result from a good balance of plant foods—plenty of nuts and peanut butter and soy bean dishes plus fruits and vegetables . . . and, remember, milk and eggs don't diminish the life of a cow or chicken. . . ."

Of course, there are other variations, but these three represent groups that are poor, have personal preferences, are satisfied with obesity, and might be referred to by health personnel on the right of the continuum as "kooky food faddists." Can the health education messages be geared to their values? Should they be?

DRINKING OF ALCOHOLIC BEVERAGES is another arena for potential value variation. Health education's dominant values are more apt to be : (1) do not drink; (2) if you drink, do not get drunk; and

(3) do not drive after drinking. Variants from the right of the continuum follow:

Variant	Possible Response
"No drinking at all should be tolerated. Alcohol is a liquid narcotic that kills brain cells with every drink and turns men and women into barbarous animals. People who drink deserve all the harm that comes to them . . . and more."	"No drinking at all is certainly the safest behavior . . . but a fair, objective look at those who drink probably does not show most drinkers as barbarous animals. When dislike of a behavior turns to vindictiveness, one must question if that is healthy behavior."
"I like to drink and I like to get drunk. I work hard most of the time. . . . I'm a responsible . . . even compulsively proper person. But then I like to 'tie one on'. . . and get really drunk. I say, and my friends agree, that I never get sloppy or nasty . . . just witty, loose . . . even occasionally brave and foolhardy."	"There are safe ways and dumb ways to drink to drunkenness. One important thing is to be with friends, particularly some who don't get drunk. After a certain 'feel good' point, drinking more will make you feel worse . . . learn from your bad nights as well as your good ones."

In these instances, one variant was toward an ultra-safe behavior, which resulted in some loss of best functioning in other dimensions of living. Admitting that there are safer ways to do unsafe things is a possibility and a challenge for health education.

DIAGNOSIS AND TREATMENT OF DEPARTURES FROM HEALTH. Secular health education is tempted to put down spiritual approaches to regaining health. Working from some common grounds is another possible and potentially healthy educational strategy. The dominant values can be stated as: (1) diagnosis and decisions about appropriate treatment should be made by a licensed physician or dentist; (2) treatment is based on scientific understanding of cause and effect— physical ailments typically require physical remedies, and mental problems require mental therapy. The religious point of view is listed as the variant below. A possible common ground response is in the right hand column.

Variant	Possible Response
"Disease and illness are real. They are caused either by evil forces or by God Himself in order to test a person. God is the only Healer, but He often uses certain 'special servants' to whom He gives the gift of healing. Healing comes through faith and prayer . . . but only if God wills it."	"There are various ways one can define evil. Physicians and dentists simply have other terms. God can use all kinds of healers. He certainly uses trained doctors to bring about many cures. He works in normal as well as spectacular ways."

"Departures from health are not real, but outward manifestations of a lack of proper relationships with God. Restore that relationship through prayer and reading, and health returns. We Christian Scientists may, under severe conditions, obtain medical care, but what is done does not bring about healing . . . this comes only from restoring the right relationship."

"You Christian Scientists are very willing to read and learn about life. If Christ were a scientist he certainly would take the scientific position of being willing to try something that has worked in other similar situations. If it is the relationship that is important . . . fine. Having medical or dental care too should not harm the restoration of relationships."

IN THE REALM OF SEXUALITY the dominant values would seem to be (1) premarital sexual intercourse, because it can result in a number of problems, is not recommended; (2) if intercourse does occur, pregnancy and venereal disease should be prevented; (3) if an unwanted pregnancy occurs, a safe legal abortion is preferable to an illegal one and perhaps to an unwanted child; (4) if venereal disease is contracted it should be treated early and medically. The variations on these values are many—in the direction of more control and the punishment of sex acts, in the direction of real female-male equality, and in the direction of values that accept the inevitability of sexual acts, many of which will be exploitative. Since this is not a book on sexuality, some readers may feel that sexual examples are already in abundance . . . perhaps redundance. Those who do not feel so are invited to mentally construct some variants, with appropriate healthy messages.

IN TEACHING-LEARNING . . . NEED FOR BACKGROUND. There also are some variant values when it comes to the actual teaching-learning process, particularly in the classroom setting. One value that dominates for most teachers would be a perspective on present and future from their own learning experiences—you have to have some background . . . to know and understand certain things before good health decisions can be made. In the extreme, this value translates to memorizing bones and muscles before considering exercise, learning all the parts and functions of the digestive tract before considering anything about food selection and eating patterns, and, of course, being able to accurately tag the epididymis and the vas deferens before dealing with any aspects of sexual behavior. Without a teacher's perspective, some learners, in effect, say, "I see no point in that tedious task" and may be completely "turned off" when the time comes to make the application to the behavior of people. By the time the alveoli can be accurately differentiated from the esophagus, there may be no time for a decision-making discussion on smoking. If the teacher, on the other hand, is concerned that students be motivated to learn about their health, she/he may employ the value that, in considering the merits of psychotherapy vs. drug therapy for mental illness, learners come to realize they need to know some things about the nervous and endocrine system. This is the more appropriate way to get background information.

Some teachers still reflect a bit of Puritan heritage, where learning was supposed to be hard and dreary and learners had to be forced to learn. Some students still reflect this heritage—a course is not a good one unless it is difficult. If the culture and its youngsters hold this value, the system works with a fairly high failure rate. However, those advocating and carrying on the system are the relative successes. But if other values prevail, as in American culture at this time, this approach will not result in learning for some youngsters. If learning is the desired product for as many as possible, then other values need to be tried. For students who have to have some personally valid reason for learning something, an approach that starts from "where they are". . . with their own experiences . . . is more likely to produce learning.

SEQUENCE OF LESSONS. Another dominant teacher value, embodied in most curricula, is symbolized by the announcement, "Today we are beginning a two-week unit on oral health." The value: it is good to develop a sequence of lessons that build a concept, each class section based on previous ones and leading to subsequent activities. Maximum learning thus comes, most typically, to students who attend the class regularly, have an attention span that encompasses the total class session, and possess the ability, natural and developed, to tie each day's activities with the other day's instructions—i.e., to think like the teacher does. For learners who do not value regular attendance or disciplined attention or who see no need to develop concepts based on relationships, the two-week unit can be a real loser.

Two possible alternatives seem feasible. One would design each day's learning activity to be complete and have integrity in and of itself. It could relate to ones before and after, but this is not necessary. It allows regular, attentive students to build larger concepts, but it can also involve and help the youngster who happens to be there . . . or awake . . . on any day. Another alternative would have one large focal concept for a whole semester or year, with all learning relating to it, though not necessarily on a day-to-day basis.

ACTION MAKES A DIFFERENCE? Finally, a fundamental value behind health education is the belief that taking action can make a difference in what happens in the future. Probably the most difficult variant value to confront, then, is one on inaction, stemming from the belief that doing something rarely makes any difference . . . that the individual really cannot affect his/her future in positive, predictable ways.

Is there any legitimate way to carry on health education without trying to change this value? Most would say NO . . . that the raison d'être of health education is to urge people to realize they have or may have problems, and that there are ways to solve and prevent such departures from full functioning. Nevertheless, given the presumption of this chapter . . . it may be important to devise health education for human beings other than those with the culture's dominant values.

We have not really dealt with particular groups in the population who hold variations of some of the culture's dominant values, mostly because the total situation is almost too complex to write about. Some black Americans affirm with conviction that there are some clearly black values that white people cannot share. Other black people deny this . . . or find it hard to clearly state such values. Some black people live with one pattern of values and then work, with whites, employing a pattern somewhat different. Are a black woman's values more predominantly black . . . or female . . . if these are not consistent? Some young people espouse values other than those of their parents. A few seem to try to live these out in adult life, but many eventually follow patterns more like their upbringing.

Perhaps it is important to pose two very general categories of people who do not hold what are considered to be dominant values. There are two dangers in such a hypothesis, however: (1) Americans today are unlikely to be consistent . . . a group may uphold some dominant values and reject others . . . and each individual in the group is likely to have some different pattern of allegiance and belief than each other member; and (2) any particular value is not held on an all-or-none basis . . . two people may value flossing the teeth in addition to brushing, but one does it regularly and the other very sporadically. And the variations are endless. So this seemingly dichotomous categorization may be futile . . . even infuriating. But you won't know till I offer it . . . so. . . .

. . . People, mostly youth and young adults, have grown up with many of the dominant cultural values, but have rejected some of them for a counter culture. These folk tend to be relatively homogeneous with an amalgam of values, some of which are clearly counter to the dominant pattern and some of which are purifications (e.g., settling differences, internationally even, by negotiation rather than by force, or war).

. . . There are people, of all ages, who have never lived by the dominant values, mainly because of low and erratic economic functioning and/or other ethnic preferences. These folk are a very heterogeneous lot, groups often being as unlike one another as they are unlike the dominant culture (i.e., Blacks in Harlem, Chicanos in East Los Angeles, whites in the Appalachians, and Blackfeet Indians in Idaho).

The major difference would be that people who have grown up with certain values and then have rejected some of them have less difficulty falling back to conformity with such than those who have grown up without them. For example:

- Willard was raised to learn and practice self-control, putting up with frustration and working out problems. He learned through life at home that alcohol use was moderate and drug use only for special, medically-prescribed purposes. As a late teenager, he chucked all these values and made the "whole drug scene" for about four years. After a close call with an overdose, he took stock of life, left the "scene," and entered college. He is now preparing for a career in pharmacy, having reaccepted most of the values of his early home life without much difficulty.

- Ben grew up in a different family setting with early remembrances of older people taking pills and drinking to excess. He grew up trying all kinds of dope, because life wasn't very shiny and promising when you were straight or sober. He is a bright boy and he has a chance to get some further education and move out of this environment. However, when things get frustrating, he finds it almost impossible not to get away from it all with a pill or a drink.

So, there has not been much attempt here to identify particular racial, economic or ethnic groups and particular variations on health issues uniquely characteristic of them . . . for the valid reasons already expressed. It might be wise, then, to leave it at that.

A SUMMARY.

- Americans, as individuals who are also part of certain groups, vary considerably in the values they hold. Perhaps health education needs to consider what its content and process would be in other than the dominant value mold.

- Eating patterns, use of alcoholic beverages, and treatment of departures from health are samples of health-related areas where variations from the dominant values are presently evident.

- The needs for background and for a sequence of related lessons are examples of values that teachers have that may thwart learning by some youngsters.

- The value on inaction, stemming from the belief that taking action rarely makes a forseeable difference, is probably the hardest value for health education not to try to change.

- Two different bases for variation from dominant values are (1) had them, but rejected them, and (2) never had them; perhaps never wanted them.

SOME KIND OF CONCLUSION. Though American culture is awash with variations on values, there are certain discernible DOMINANT values, some of which are expressed fairly vividly in health textbooks. Yet there are some health educators who feel that if their profession is to communicate with and motivate all to better health—rather than just those with the dominant values—we must consider the merit of a position allowing almost any behavior as long as it helps a person function. But how does health education come across when one accepts the variants in values? Rather strange . . . perhaps threatening. But it may be important to try to meet needs that we have neglected.

And we are people with a high value on trying . . . on setting out to accomplish what needs doing. It is thus hard to know what to do with an insight from Zen Buddhism . . . you achieve what is worthwhile by not striving for it . . . and you cannot strive to not strive.

Chapter XI

Curriculum Development

You have in your hands the text for this Health course, *This Is Your Healthy Life*. It has eighteen chapters, and there are eighteen weeks in the semester. We'll cover one chapter each week, in order. I'll assign the reading for you to do each night, and we'll reread it in class the next day. We'll have discussion if there is time, but we need to cover the assigned material. Each Friday, there will be a true-false test over the week's chapter, and there will be a true-false examination over the whole book at the end of the semester.

This is basic, tried-and-true curriculum, used in more or less perfect form by some teachers at all levels. This approach has some real advantages or it obviously would not still be employed.

1. The content and the sequence have been determined by experts, i.e., the text writer or writers.

2. The time to be given to each topic is determined in a simple fashion: there are eighteen weeks and eighteen chapters—one per week.

3. The objectives are simple: students will learn everything they can from a chapter each week.

4. The teaching-learning approach is simple, not confusing, and one that students can feel comfortable with—because there is no deviation; reading the book at home and then rereading it aloud in class reinforces what it says, does not add extraneous, confusing facts or ideas, and is the most direct way to achieve the objective.

5. The teacher retains control of the class so that there are no interruptions in the learning process. The teacher and the book are the final authorities, giving feelings of security to the class.

6. All students have equal access to the learning resource—the book.

7. Evaluation is consistent and fair, because it does not penalize students who do not express themselves well or who are not creative. With a standard number of points each week that accumulate in a predictable way, and with no other influences on the grade, each student knows exactly where she/he stands at any time.

Sounds rather ideal, doesn't it? For some, this is a sufficient statement about curriculum, its development and its implications. I am not going to agree. . . . As you see, this chapter is considerably longer. It is important to see this as basic curriculum and have some justifications ready for going beyond it. The first such justification is that the American ethic is to look for ever better ways to accomplish anything . . . and there may be better ways to learn more . . . or to achieve different goals . . . or to learn differently.

So, let us start in another way . . . first, the general and philosophical:

- Curriculum must exist within a framework of philosophical assumptions about the dignity and worth of human beings.

Then, becoming more specific:

- Curriculum consists of both content and process.

An amplification of the first statement would be:

- Curriculum is an organized approach to learning content through selected processes.

Extending this amplification:

- Curriculum is a purposeful organized approach to learning content through selected processes.

Further amplification:

- Curriculum is a purposeful organized approach to learning concepts, facts, ideas . . . through learning activities that are effectively described.

Still further:

- Curriculum is a purposeful organized approach to learning concepts, facts, ideas . . . through learning activities that are effectively described, including learning resources of various kinds, which are listed, described, and available.

And finally:

- Curriculum is a purposeful organized approach to learning concepts, facts, ideas . . . through learning activities that are effectively described, including learning resources of various kinds, which are listed, described, and available, and including descriptions of a number of ways to determine to what extent the purposes of the learning were achieved.

In short, curriculum within a philosophical framework consists of
A Philosophy of Health Education
    Objectives
        Content Material
           Learning Activities
              Resource Materials
                Evaluation Procedures

But before developing each of these more fully than you may want to consider, muse on this perspective.

The classroom teacher—or the educator who actually works with the learners in the learning setting, whatever it may be—develops actual curriculum. Actual curriculum is what actually happens. True curriculum can be described only in retrospect. Much of this chapter will be about that which attempts to influence the teacher before she/he does what she/he actually does.

THE CONTENT OF CURRICULUM. Curriculum is both content and process. Our first concern here will be with content, or what curriculum is. It probably would be logical to start with objectives, but this is not the only possible starting point. Curriculum development could begin with some methods of evaluation . . . with some excellent resource materials . . . with some effective ways to learn . . . or with some important facts, ideas, and concepts. The crucial point is not with what one begins, but rather whether all of the elements are finally tied together effectively. That is, the content is related directly to the objective, the learning activities are all possible ways of helping learners achieve the objective, the resource materials are related to both the content and the learning activities, and the evaluation procedures really can determine to what extent the objective has been accomplished.

In Chapter II, you read a brief description of three philosophies of education, emphasizing that each one views the teaching task differently. Likewise with curriculum. The major concern of the realist is with the content material—the knowledge to be learned. The experimentalist is more interested in the learning activities and the evaluation —what learners are doing to create knowledge and what they are doing to give evidence of active learning. The idealist might have some concern about resource materials, but she/he would show the least interest in the curriculum plan, feeling that the personal influence of the teacher (relatively unfettered by a plan) is the truly important factor in students' learning.

Traditionally, the content has been the most important element in the curriculum—hence the reason for the textbook being the basic curriculum. The content is most important when the knowledge in a field can be expected to hold true and steady for the lifetime of the learner—when what a youngster learns at age 15 is likely to be true when she/he is 35, 55, even 75. When there is less assurance that knowledge will stay constant, then the process, or learning how to learn, rises in import. There need to be fewer statements like, "We all learned the Seven Basic Food Groups, and I don't think I'll ever forget them," "We learned about TB and why they have to have all those special sanitoriums," and "We learned that hospitalization for mental illness is very important, so we have to have more mental hospitals."

There may need to be more learning activity statements such as:

We read some accounts of tuberculosis treatment thirty years ago and some about today . . . now we're developing the script for a short film that would dramatize these clear differences in treatment style.

I was working with this group . . . there were four of us . . . and we experimented with putting food into two basic groups and on up to ten groups. We could see why in the past there were seven groups, and we saw the merits of more groups and fewer. I don't think I could have done it alone, but we all benefitted from the ideas each of the four of us had . . . and so came to trust each other to say things we might have been afraid to say just in a pick-up group.

I've really learned how to research a topic, going from one bibliography to another. In mental health treatment, I can see how we've moved out of the era of just hospital care, and it's fascinating to read the speculations about innovations in community treatment methods for the future.

In a broader sense, the learner of today probably needs to be impressed less with the "facts the book gave and the teacher repeated" and more with "I thought everyone would interpret it the way I did, but the discussion showed that there were several other defensible ways of looking at it." Health teaching probably should encourage the open mind as well as encouraging a good, solid, intellectual content.

THREE DOMAINS. When I first learned something about the health curriculum, I learned that there were three focuses for learning—knowledge, attitudes, and practices. Contemporary curriculum terminology refers to these as the cognitive domain, the affective domain, and the action domain.[1,2,3,4] However it is phrased, it means what you know, how you feel about what you know, and what you do about what you know. The curriculum must address itself to these three domains in some way.

---

[1] Bloom, Benjamin S. (Ed.), *Taxonomy of Educational Objectives, Handbook I: Cognitive Domain.* New York: David McKay Co., Inc., 1956.

[2] Krathwohl, David R., Bloom, Benjamin S., and Masia, Bertram B., *Taxonomy of Educational Objectives, Handbook II: Affective Domain.* New York: David McKay Co., Inc., 1964.

[3] The third Handbook in the Taxonomy series was to be on the Psychomotor Domain. It was not published. The School Health Education Study utilized the first two domains plus the idea inherent in the third, but changed the terminology to the Action Domain.

[4] School Health Education Study Writing Group, *Health Education: A Conceptual Approach to Curriculum Design.* St. Paul: 3M Education Press, 1967. pg. 26.

MANY INFLUENCES. Ideally, the curriculum emerges from a balance of influences and inputs . . . on both content and process.

- The subject field reports all that there is possible to know— typically much more than any learner or class could comfortably deal with. Learning theorists, educational researchers, and practical pedogogical journals provide many new ways of encouraging learning. Both health and education professionals share the task of deciding scope and sequence—when certain content should be introduced, how often and when it should be repeated, and how one area of learning can lead to another. Content may be part of the development of concepts, which will be dealt with more extensively later.

- The community in which a school is located feeds in both desirable topics and learning, and restrictions on what will be dealt with and how.

In one community, parents and non-parents, professionals and non-professionals seem to agree that a study of mental health at the ninth-grade level should get down to the concerns of students in the class and that methods of working out problems should be stimulated in the classroom, utilizing trained guidance help. In a community not too far away, certain influential community members would call such a curriculum item sensitivity training, a plot to undermine the character and morals of youth, and neither the content nor the methodology would dare be included.

The age group, sex and other general characteristics of the students in a class will often influence curriculum. Such statements as these give evidence of this influence:

"Kids of this age need to learn about. . . ."
"Kids in this grade are really interested in. . . ."
"Girls will be interested in . . . but most boys won't."
"That may be all right for your comfortable suburban school, but my kids need to deal with . . . in more plain, open language."

Finally, to the extent that she/he can and wants to, the teacher considers the learners in a class as individuals and varies learning activities and expectations according to needs and abilities of students. The evidence:

"Cathy needs to know about contraception, but some of the other girls don't . . . at this age."

"Bill needs to read or see something in order to learn it . . . if he only hears it, not much learning is likely. . . ."

Another, somewhat more contemporary, way of organizing the content material is as concepts. Concepts are big, generalized ideas about something, summarizers of all our experiences with that phenomenon to a particular point. Woodruff[5] called a concept "the internal mediating variable that accounts for the direction of a person's response to a situation." Since perceptions contain both cognitive and affective elements, concepts have both elements also and thus mediate both rational and emotional behavior. Any concept worth the title is never completely learned. As long as a person is having any experiences, personal or academic, relating to it, the concept is being built further. Facts help build concepts, but so do experiences and analyses and evaluations of experiences. A curriculum built on concepts sends learners forth with more fully developed concepts than they would have without it, but still with much more to learn.

RESOURCE MATERIALS. The curriculum will be based on some amount of resource material. The basic, skimpiest menu was presented at the birth of this chapter: one textbook. The expansion goes to listing and describing materials presenting a wider range of ideas, facts, and viewpoints. It also includes a wider variety of types of resources. The book is basic; other books widen the possible learning; films, transparencies, pamphlets, booklets, and resource people broaden the possible learning experience. Some curricula have extra resource material merely appended. Others genuinely are based on the use of a wide, broad range of supplementary materials by students.

EVALUATION is both objective and subjective. Objective means that the teacher subjectively accepts some others' judgments and arbitrarily chooses some form of question that is correct if answered b or F or 3. The difference between subjective and objective, which is not dichotomous, is the apparent influence of the teacher's personal judgment. Another distinction in evaluation is that which is assessed for credit and that which is assessed not for credit. A teacher may say, "Karen is doing well in class," but Karen's grade is based on a single multiple choice exam and, despite her doing well, she gets a low C on her grade card. How well is Karen doing, anyway? To highlight the opposite: I remember one year having two pole vaulters, Walter and George. Afternoon practices were periodically shattered by the sound of wooden crossbars splintering. Yet, however many crossbars were reduced to kindling during the week, when both Walter and George went past 11 feet on Saturday and placed first and second . . . the evaluation had to be positive because they showed they had learned when it counted.

Another critical aspect of evaluation that the curriculum may direct is the amount of competition against others versus the amount of competition with self alone.

---

[5] Woodruff, Asahel D., "The Use of Concepts in Teaching and Learning," *The Journal of Teacher Education*, March 1964, pg. 84.

Students will be ranked according to demonstrated knowledge of the cycle of infection and the number of disease examples accurately described. Extra points will be given those top ten who can describe the most diseases.

or

The standard is set up . . . anyone can reach it . . . if all succeed, all get A's.

OBJECTIVES, AT LAST. Remember . . . it was logical to begin with objectives, but the notion was superseded by one that it is possible to build curriculum starting with any element. So we seem to have all the elements except the objectives. Better last than not at all. The simplest form of objctive is one dealing only with content . . . with what the student will know after some learning experiences. Such an objective often employs the verb "understands," leaving it up to the teacher to decide to what extent students understand. Such an objective might be:

Understands the nature of food fads and fallacies

It might be accompanied by an attitudinal objective such as:

Appreciates the dangers of food fads and fallacies

A semi-behavioral objective begins with a verb that gives the teacher a bit more direction as to what appropriate learning and evaluation activities might be, but still gives the educators leeway in selecting exactly how to teach and in deciding whether it has been accomplished. Such an objective might sound like:

Distinguishes between food fads, fallacies, and diets based on scientific principles of nutrition

This leaves many options for how students are to "distinguish between."

A behavioral objective, finally, is concerned with what learners are to do and, particularly, with what they are to accomplish. An example:

Students are able to distinguish between food fads and fallacies and sound nutrition practices on a recognition, matching type instrument with 70 percent accuracy and are able to write at least four accurate distinctions from memory.

BEHAVIORAL OBJECTIVES come out of the programmed learning movement, and, therefore, are based on the assumption that all learners will accomplish the objective, which will require more time for some, less time for others. Where this kind of flexibility and individual rates of progress are not possible—or desired by the teacher—the objective could be seen as the criterion for a C grade (or B or A), with those accomplishing more receiving higher grades and those accomplishing less lower grades.

Behavioral objectives are part of the contemporary movement for accountability—to be more certain as to what students are and are not learning. But behavioral objectives are constructed on the premise that all significant learning can be quantified and measured . . . or, said the other way, that what cannot be quantified and measured is not worth trying to learn. Behavioral objectives were defended by Popham[6] in 1968, with the following major points:

1. Behavioral objectives indicate what the teacher is going to have students do. If they are trivial, then the learning will be trivial. The teacher who is going to have students deal with important ideas in meaningful ways can state this in the form of an objective or objectives.

2. Behavioral objectives are directions for achieving pupil growth. If unique instructional opportunities arise and the teacher deviates from the objective, it is important to see whether or not this departure achieved growth—or was only a temporary diversion, Spontaneous learning activities, too, need to be justified.

3. There may be other important social outcomes from school, but its primary responsibility is to encourage youngsters to learn. Behavioral objectives indicate what the student hopefully will do and will attain.

4. All valid measurement is not done by multiple-choice and true-false tests. These are ways in which people assess complicated human behavior, and these can be translated into objectives.

5. Having behavioral objectives does not make a teacher insensitive to the unanticipated opportunities for learning, but does give her/him something more tangible and direct from which to deviate. They tend to discourage too frequent deviation from the planned and specified.

THE THREE DOMAINS AGAIN. The objectives of health education traditionally have been in three realms—knowledge, attitudes, and practices. In the terminology of the curriculum movement, the objectives need to be in the cognitive, affective, and action domains. Cognitive objectives can be put in behavioral form fairly easily and lend themselves to checking in the classroom. However, as I attempt to write a

---

[6] Popham, W. James, "Probing the Validity of Arguments Against Behavioral Goals," Symposium Presentation at American Educational Research Association Meeting, February 1968.
and
    Popham, W. James, *Educational Objectives.* Los Angeles: Vincent Associates, 1966.

behavioral objective, I find that they seem to develop easiest with the least important information.

Students will be able to list, in order, the six steps in the chain of infection.

Health education is big on attitudes, and we talk a lot about modifying and improving attitudes, but as we construct a behavioral objective we're struck with two dilemmas: (1) Do we really want all students to feel exactly the same? Can we say Susan has not achieved the objective if her attitude varies from the objective? and (2) most health attitudes will be displayed in life situations other than the classroom. What a youngster says she/he will feel like if_____happens may or may not be accurate. Let's try a few:

Students will feel mild disgust with a person becoming intoxicated, and the disgust will increase in intensity as the intoxication becomes more marked.

Students will feel pity for the person suffering from the illness of alcoholism.*

Students will admire people who drive carefully and under the speed limit.

As noted, none of these are likely to be measurable in the classroom. And because they are evidenced in some degree in association with a wide variety of people in different situations—and, along with many other attitudes—they are not necessarily going to be felt consistently.

If all this is true of attitudes, it certainly is true of practices, behavior . . . the objectives in the action domain. Namely, they are not susceptible to measurement in the classroom. A good behavior objective that would certainly prevent all drunkenness would be:

A student will never consume more than ½ ounce of ethyl alcohol in any beverage or drink in a one hour period.

Another form is less easy to measure, but specifies some of the behavioral reasoning behind the recommended practice:

The student avoids the use of substances that modify mood and behavior in amounts that reduce the ability to think clearly and react normally.

CONCLUSIONS ON OBJECTIVES. How does it all sum up? Objectives give the direction for the teaching-learning experience. They indicate a plan and a goal. They can be very exact, very behavioral . . . or they can be very general. Some teachers are very conscious of objectives, and some appear not to be. I have seen no research attempt-

---

* These two illustrate one of our health ambivalences—you can hate and castigate the drunk, but when he/she becomes an alcoholic, then you should love and feel compassion for him/her.

ing to correlate any elements of success in teaching with awareness of objectives. I would hypothesize a slight correlation, but nothing startling. Some excellent teachers have objectives internalized . . . they just know what they're trying to accomplish. But a poor teacher without conscious objectives can be a disaster. One personal note and suggestion: I believe in objectives and use them consciously in my teaching. My advice to myself and to other teachers, in-service or pre-service education is: if for any reason you decide to deviate from the planned objective for a class, honestly translate what you actually did into an objective and see how it sounds. It might read

> Students should be able to air strong feelings about school, teachers, teaching methods, and class atmosphere, when provoked by a run-in with a previous teacher and the unrest of a windy blustery afternoon

or

> Students profit from listening to the teacher tell stories of her/his youth, most of which have nothing to do with the subject matter for the course.

Each may be defensible once in a while, but are they as worthy as what was planned?

HOW CURRICULUM COMES TO BE. Curriculum is a product. Curriculum development is a process. How is a curriculum devised? One simple way opened this chapter; the textbook is the curriculum.

Another simple one is that a knowledgeable teacher sort of makes it up as she/he goes along.

These are the bare ones. Now curriculum will be redefined as a tangible product . . . something written down . . . something to guide all teachers of health at a particular age or grade level. How can such be produced?

The simplest way is to have one knowledgeable person, say, Dr. Billings, whose writing is reasonably understandable, sit down and write the curriculum—objectives, content, teaching-learning activities, resource materials, and evaluative procedures.

There are three possible advantages to this system: (1) it tends to be of consistent style and quality; (2) it can be relatively inexpensive; (3) it can be produced and be in the hands of the teachers in a minimum period of time. The obvious difficulty is in finding this inexpensive Dr. Billings, with the time and the omniscience to be in command of content, teaching-learning approaches, and all the rest.

Another way is to form a committee of knowledgeable people who get together, delegate and accept responsibilities, and produce a group project. In the ideal, this could be a faster process than Dr. Billings' solo flight, but rarely do all the members of a committee agree or judge things in comparable ways, and rarely do all work at the same rate. There must be time for discussion, wrangling, and compromise (maybe even for outside resource people to settle disputes). Also, the product is produced according to the pace of the slowest member.

All of the disadvantages of these two processes are countered by the ideal curriculum development scheme, the elements of which are found in the River City K-12 Health Education Super Project.

- The project has a single administrator or a small compatibly functioning committee to direct its various operations.

- An extensive survey is done of all relevant sources for objectives— the various health-related literature, students, older students (who can look back and indicate what they would like to have learned), parents, interested elements in the community, teachers, and professional health educators.

- Resource people are selected to make recommendations on the content and its proper scope and sequence, others on the learning approaches, others on resource materials, and others on evaluation methods.

- A group is selected to do the writing, some of whom are experts in the content and some who are master teachers, all of whom have developed skill in writing. Everything written is critiqued by the whole group and rewritten to conform to the best compromise of judgments.

- Some of the resource people also do critiques of the written product, and more compromises must be reached.

Some of the decisions that must be made are:

- The style of presentation—parallel columns? Long way on the page? Space for teacher to make notes? How much in one volume? Printed or mimeographed or other?

- How much content to include? Some guides have virtually no content material, but merely contain questions that anyone teaching should be able to answer. At the other extreme . . . I worked recently in some implementation workshops for a curriculum in alcohol and alcohol safety that has 129 full pages of content material—a respectable textbook within the guide.

- How thoroughly should learning activities be described? If films or other visual materials are suggested, how thoroughly should the content be described? Should actual films be suggested? If students are to prepare a checklist, how complete is the model in the guide? If groups are to be formed, should methods of formation be explained? If individuals or groups are researching topics, how many samples should be listed or amplified? If an experiment is

to be done, how thorough should the description of materials, procedures, and evaluation be? If students are to develop a list of
factors, should a list of the kinds of items they might be expected
to come up with be included? How extensive? If students are to
develop a questionnaire or a survey form, how extensive should
the example or model be? If students are to debate, how many
possible debate topics should be listed? If students are to analyze
problems, how many should be included and how thoroughly
described should each be? If students are to role play, how
extensively are possible roles described?

WHAT DO TEACHERS WANT? Some assumption has to be made
about the sort of teacher to whom the guide is directed. One group of
teachers, whose spokesman is Papa Bear, says, "All of this detail is a
silly waste . . . they take two pages to describe role-playing . . . I
certainly know how to get kids to role play . . . most of the examples
aren't necessary." Another group, led by Mama Bear, complains,
"There just isn't enough detail. It says that students should apply
values to hypothetical situations influencing protection from disease,
which I think is a good activity, but there are only four examples given,
and I don't like two of them. How do they expect us to carry out the
activity without some more situations to choose from?" You just have
to hope that there are enough in the group for which Baby Bear speaks,
"The learning activities are described very nicely. There are examples
so you have some ideas of what the writers had in mind, but you're not
coerced into using their ideas. The examples help you develop your
own situations, applicable to your own class group.

- Somewhat akin to this above dilemma is that of how many activities to describe? If the objective is "compares potential social and
psychological values of smoking with the possible detrimental
effects," should there be one thoroughly described activity, or
three, or eight, or eleven? How many ways are there to "compare?"

- How many resources should be listed? How many should be
annotated? Should selections be made or should everything available and known be listed? Should any judgments on quality be
indicated? Is there any standard for age . . . or length of time
since publishing . . . that should be utilized?

Some guides are written for Ms. Dennis who says, "I like lots of
choices, I like more content than I can use, plenty of learning activities,
resource materials, and evaluation things from which to choose . . .
even some variety in objectives. With the same guide, I can teach
different classes in different ways."

The same guides are also given to Ms. Barton who says, "I never
saw such a confusing thing in my life. What am I expected to do . . .

cover five objectives with ten activities each? I know I'm supposed to make choices, but how do I know what is best? I wish there was more guidance given . . . and not so many choices."

And so it goes.

PROS AND CONS. The pros and cons of approaches that tend toward Dr. Billings and those toward the River City Project essentially boil down to:

Time:

- The number of months or years between the first imperative for the curriculum and the published product.
- The person-hours involved, and how many of these really hastened the development and how many impeded progress.

Money:

- Since it is rare, in this era, that curriculum is developed as a voluntary contribution of time and expertise, the item above on person-hours may translate into some amount of money that must be paid some way or other. If funds are limited, the process may have to match what is available.

Quality:

- Do classroom teachers, unaware of the method by which the curriculum was developed, see differences in quality that pragmatically, rather than theoretically, show one style superior to the other?

IMPLEMENTATION. But wait . . . the curriculum development process is not over when the manuscript is in—or even when the finished product is printed and available. Remember an earlier adage: curriculum is developed by the teacher in the classroom. Likewise, this organized, printed curriculum has not finished its development process until it influences some number of individual teachers in classrooms. This includes traditional Mrs. Finnegan, authoritative Mr. Grenwell, far-out Ms. Farmer, and many others. A curriculum makes most sense to—communicates best with—those who wrote it. Those who were not involved in this process may or may not care how it was done. If it communicates, fine . . . if not, too bad. Workshops, some in-service experiences, and good supervision often can help greatly in urging teachers to use a new curriculum. If not enough resources are put into this phase, the beauty of the product is lost.

And, to cap this off, here is a lesson I learned in this implementation process. Several years ago, I conducted a two-week workshop for a district that had adopted a health curriculum on which I had labored. There were some very creative people in the workshop groups. Toward the end, I found myself resenting the time I was spending with one of the least promising teachers in the group (in my hastily formed judgment.) How much more valuable it would be (as well as fun!) to be spending the time with the excited, interested, creative ones. But I resisted the temptation. Two years later I found out that virtually all the creative ones had left the district. The best health programs in the district were then being spearheaded by my least promising student. The next best programs were developed by a close friend of his, due to his influence. So mobility means that implementation may be a nearly continuous process. It also suggests, don't waste time making judgments about what teachers are really good. Help each as much as possible, for in a few years any one could be the mainstay of an ongoing program.

THE PRE-PROCESS. Now, let's go back a bit. This section of process began with some pure clarion call for a new health curriculum. Is this realistic? What is the process before the process? Earlier pages have indicated that health is no clearly mandated subject for all schools, that sometimes it is developed as a comprehensive K-12, general education type course. More often, however, it appears in order to deal with some recognized social problems, like venereal disease. Community support is unlikely to be massive, and even less likely, to be consistently favorable. Personalities get involved, egos and rivalries emerge. Sometimes a total curriculum is developed because of the influence of one person. In other instances, there is no curriculum because of another one person. And so with groups.

In order to deal with this process in the human form in which it occurs, I have developed a sociodrama that I utilized twice in a graduate course, "Curriculum Development in Health Education." The situation is as follows:

Let's Do Something About the Health Education Curriculum!

A Drama To Provoke Thought

Mr. Bruce Morgan, the principal of Southern High School, has called a meeting to discuss possible changes and innovations in the health education curriculum of his school.. The impetus really has come from Dr. Benson, a professor of health education at a nearby university, who has worked with two Southern High School teachers on some curriculum materials. Mr. Morgan opens the meeting . . .

Participants:

Mr. Bruce Morgan—Principal. Considers himself an educational leader, but really prides himself on being a flexible, practical administrator, seeing all sides of all issues. Mr. Morgan has taught science in junior high, but only as a stepping stone to administration; likes to see his school as modern and innovative, but realizes the practical problems of innovation; enjoys the challenge of administering change, with little concern for any particular result in learning; considers the university consultant and the curriculum director impractical, but realizes it is politically necessary to have them present; considers health education a legitimate off-shoot of physical education; considers that it would be mostly information-giving rather than involving much discussion; all his department chairmen are men—he feels that men should make the decisions in a school.

Ms. Henrietta (Mr. Henry) Rasmussen—Curriculum Director for the High School District. He/she is very much committed to Bruner's theory of instruction and has worked on one of the first mathematics projects based on concept learning; he/she is convinced that this type of teaching-learning can be more exciting and produce better results; he/she believes that administrators should provide the time for teachers to be educated in new methods; he/she views health as watered-down science.

Dr. Robert (Roberta) Benson—University Consultant and Professor of Health Education. Strong advocate of the Concept Approach to health teaching; does not see health education as a string of problems; realizing that all subject matter cannot be covered, he/she advocates emphasis on process—on developing a way of thinking about health, with continual attention to the dynamic interrelationships among the physical, mental-emotional, and social dimensions; he/she encourages adolescents to make many of their own decisions and to examine these decisions in the learning environment; would like to see health education considered separate from and equal to physical education.

"Big Ed" Rowan—Chairman of Health and Physical Education for Boys and Girls. A physical education major and ex-coach; concerned with what he considers a proper balance among health education, physical education, and athletics; believes major responsibility is to provide activity for sedentary adolescents; uses the district's fact-oriented curriculum guide in health; views curriculum as content, with the Guide and a textbook as sufficient.

Dr. Frank (or Frances) Dewer—a local private physician, an internist specializing in adolescent problems. Prevention-oriented, but also strongly problem-oriented; feels that drinking, accidents, drug use, pregnancy, and venereal disease are the major youth problems and that a health education course should help prevent these; thinks such a program needs more medical consultation; believes physicians should give the information in large assemblies or classes and then have attitudes shaped in the smaller class sessions; sees little need for any newfangled curriculum; believes kids need to be told what is right and what is wrong.

Most of the roles can be played either by a woman or a man. The principal's instructions are to carry on the curriculum meeting until it no longer seems productive, and then to schedule a second meeting for a week later, with some possible assignments. The characters next week are all played by different people. Sometimes the prospects for the curriculum look good, sometimes fairly hopeless. And you just never know what the human factors will be. Once Dr. Benson actually got "Big Ed" to support the idea. Sometimes Dr. Dewer cooperates, sometimes he/she does not. It seems like an excellent process for becoming aware of the process of how curriculum gets developed . . . or does not.

TWO EXAMPLES OF CURRICULUM PROJECTS. The School
Health Education Study was a uniquely funded and theoretically excellent health curriculum project of the recent past, and I describe it from
the vantage point of one of the writers.

Prior to beginning the curriculum development process, the Study
produced two important documents. *Synthesis of Research in . . .
Health Instruction*[7] (a cooperative effort between the American Alliance for Health, Physical Education and Recreation and the Study)
was first published in May 1963, edited by Professor Harold Veenker
of Purdue University. Each of its first chapters was written by a different health education professional. *A Summary Report*[8] of the attitudes
and behavior came out in June 1964. With these and inputs from other
projects in the curriculum movement of the 1960's and from other
health education groups working with concepts, the writing group (six
writers, the director, and the coordinator) began to struggle with the
question of how topic-oriented or how concept-oriented the Study's
project should be. The research synthesis and the Status Study revealed
few conceptual approaches. Evidence showed that a new approach in
health education might be an improvement. The continual struggle
always came back to what is best for learners, but two other competing
forces ever present were, How will it be accepted by leaders in the
curriculum development movement? and How will it be accepted by
classroom teachers?

The writers were selected as people with the potential to generate
and actually write a curriculum. Some diversity was necessary, but too
much would have made the many necessary compromises too bloody
and time consuming. All were competent and assertive people. Each
fought hard for his/her view and compromised when necessary. When
the outside Editor and his staff were added, decisions were often even
harder.

THE FIRST GUIDES. The first teaching-learning guides were written
with the direct help of the classroom teachers from the four try-out
centers, public schools in four separate geographic areas of the United
States. This process produced a guide for each of four levels for two
concepts, a total of eight in all. This was a good process, but quite
costly in time and person-hours. The guides were used in the try-out
center schools[9] during the Spring of 1965. Pre- and post-evaluations
were carried out, gathering objective data and subjective feelings. It

---

[7] Veenker, C. Harold (Ed.), *Synthesis of Research in Selected Areas of
Health Instruction.* Washington, D.C.: School Education Study, 1963. 192 pp.

[8] Sliepcevich, Elena, *School Health Education Study: A Summary Report.*
Washington, D.C.: School Health Education Study, 1964. 74 pp.

[9] School Health Education Study Writing Group, *Health Education*, pp. 118-
119.

simply was not possible to control all of the variables in real public school settings to create a respectable research design. Further, the teachers acted as teachers rather than as participants in a research enterprise, and modified objectives and learning opportunities as it seemed best to do in the classroom. Visitations were made and extensive interviews were conducted. The central finding was that the teachers generally were excited about the conceptual approach, frustrated that they did not understand and implement it better, but eager to develop it further the next year. Much credit for the success of the development of the conceptual approach goes to these teachers.

SUBSEQUENT GUIDES. The development of subsequent guides had gone ahead while the evaluations were being made. As findings became evident, they were incorporated in the developing materials. The scope of the S.H.E.S. project—full development of ten concepts, each at four levels—when meshed with the time schedule of funding, seemed to necessitate a less participative process in producing the remaining eight sets of guides. Fundamentally, one writer was responsible for a total concept. She/he had to arrange and utilize assistance in writing and consultations of various kinds. Then the Washington office directed rewriting and editing, which was repeated with another perspective, at the publishers. The first guides were available in attractive published form in 1967. The last, equally attractive, became part of the field's curriculum literature in the fall of 1972.

NO TEXTBOOK. Guides to the first seven concepts published were supplemented by sets of visual transparencies, typically twenty per behavioral objective—approximately 400 per concept or about 100 per level per concept. Some of these were designed to be factual, some provocative of discussion, some speculative, some symbolic. . . . The key decision by the Study and the publishers to present visual transparencies as the major supplement to the curriculum rather than textbooks fit the idealistic vision of the needs of teachers in the future. Accompanying each guide at each level was an extensive listing of teacher-student resources relevant to the concept. With as many as 100 pages, these resources listed books, monographs, and reports; articles from professional journals and magazines; case studies; annotated listings of films, filmstrips, slides, scripts, tapes, transparencies, and other media. The vision was that teachers would use unique combinations of these resources (including the transparencies directly designed to help develop the Concept) rather than a single, basic textbook. This was based on the vision that school boards would see health courses without assigned textbooks as a significant, positive educational innovation and would be willing to put comparable monies into the varied resource materials.

WEAKNESSES. Two major weaknesses emerged from the School Health Education Study experience. One was the obvious need for implementation experiences to insure that basically sound guides with many choices of creative learning opportunities finally came to guide actual learning in actual classrooms. This is time consuming and expensive, and requires follow-up and refollow-up, but without it many teachers find it difficult to see the value in the guides. . . .

1. The guiding rationale of the study was that it was not to pose as a national curriculum—a fixed recipe for success in every hamlet, suburb, and metropolis.

2. The weakness is one of choice: "How in the world do we know what to select? Do we cover only certain concepts? If so, which ones? What behavioral objectives? How many learning opportunities for each? With our limited time, should we deal with fewer concepts and be more assured that most students develop them . . . or should we cover as many of these important concepts as possible?

3. The strength is "It gives us an opportunity to develop our own curriculum that fits our needs very closely."

WHERE TO NOW? The School Health Education Study made an important contribution to health curriculum development, and many adaptations have appeared. The trend now seems to be toward state, county, district and local level development of new materials. Federal funds have been available for certain limited scope projects. The early 1970's were a time of considerable funding for drug education, VD, and other special topical curriculums and projects. Less visible is support for comprehensive health education.

A SECOND CURRICULUM EXAMPLE. The "Elementary School Health Education Project"[10] is an interesting development in that it was (1) of limited scope (fifth, sixth, and seventh grades); (2) was developed through Federal funds—a three-year contract from the National Clearinghouse for Smoking and Health with the San Ramon Unified School District and the Berkeley School District in California; and (3) now has spread to many districts in various states with Clearinghouse support. The emphasis in the curriculum is on developing understanding and appreciation of the body and skills for prevention of disease, along with encouraging of youth to make their own sound decisions about personal and environmental factors that affect health. The curriculum consists of three intensive units, each to last eight to ten weeks. The fifth-grade unit centers on the lungs and the respiratory

---

10 Davis, Roy L., "New Models for Health Curriculum and Teacher Training," *School Health Review*, 5:33-36 (no. 4), July-August, 1974.

system, the sixth grade on the heart and the circulatory system, and the seventh grade on the brain and the nervous system. Regional training centers were funded, with several teacher-training institutions also competent to train for the Model. Carefully developed and sequentially arranged sets of materials were developed and supplied to the training centers. Spread of this model is dependent on perceived success, its communication to other districts, and the willingness and ability of these to provide the funds for the necessary implementation. And that is the external "rub!"

ATMOSPHERES FOR LEARNING. Another important trend is toward creating atmospheres for learning in classrooms before being concerned about curriculum. Of course, curriculum can be developed to help create warm, accepting atmospheres of learning, but often these atmospheres can be nurtured only by reacting to situations as they arise spontaneously. These are inherently anti-curriculum forces, and the rise of any strong curriculum movement is apt to stir the forces that are the antithesis of order, planning, systematic evaluation, and predictability.

IN SUMMARY.

- The most basic curriculum is the textbook, with reading, reciting, learning, and testing based on it.
- Curriculum and curriculum development both involve content and process—what and how.
- The curriculum emerges from a balance of many influences and inputs—the subject field, the learners, and the community.
- Curriculum arises from some philosophy of health education; functionally, it consists of objectives, content, learning activities, evaluation procedures, and resource materials.
- Health curricula must deal with the cognitive (knowledge), affective (attitudes) and action (behavior) domains.
- The curriculum development process can range from very simple to exceedingly complex.
- Not all teachers emphasize the same thing in the development of curriculum.
- The School Health Education Study was a nationally oriented, K-12, comprehensive health curriculum developed through complex, but theoretically sound, processes.
- The Elementary School Health Education Project uses a crisis problem—smoking as a basis for learning about the body, making decisions, and forming attitudes.

- Present trends are toward local adaptations, more limited grade levels, or special problem units, representing another portion of the curriculum cycle.

- Atmospheres for learning are inherent forces opposing ordered curriculum development.

- In recognition of the relationships between health behavior, health problems, and health status, many states are legislating comprehensive health education statutes.

Chapter XII

Teaching-Learning Strategies

One Basic Strategy Focuses on

Better Teaching

Another Basic Strategy Focuses on

More and Better Learning

"Now, that is silly! These are not antithetical . . . good instruction certainly results from a balance of each."

As much as I like syntheses and eclectic conclusions, this still seems to me to be a matter of different—even diametric—emphasis. The goal of the first is a strong teacher, the acknowledged font of learning . . . the source . . . the final authority . . . the one who has learned, who now seeks to teach others . . . the guru who responds as learners need help with vexing questions and ambiguities. The goal of the second, as I see it, is a strong, confident director of learning . . . one who still considers her/himself a learner, first and foremost . . . one who would prefer to guide a student to a source of information that can be revisited, rather than provide it her/himself . . . one less concerned with the fact that something is clearly authoritative and more with how useful it is or what it means . . . one who facilitates learning and quietly supervises and guides it without dominance. In other words, in one strategy the one who knows, tells. In the other, the one who knows would rather learners developed other ways of knowing rather than simply listening to him/her.

If we should review the three basic philosophies of education in this context, in my view, we may be struck with the sense that in:

- *Idealism* the teacher is most important. Communication and learning are a matter of minds in tune. There really are no necessary strategies of teaching-learning; the learner's constant association with the teacher is the critical factor.

- *Realism* the teacher is a purveyor of knowledge, but may be assisted by the text, content films, other books, other resources, etc. Knowledge is where you find it, and the teacher has some, but needs to know where else to find it available to students.

- *Experimentalism* each learner creates knowledge on his/her own from active processes; the teacher is one who encourages youngsters to learn and guides them in a variety of repeatable ways, interested that they learn how to learn. Knowledge is created.

IMPRESSIONS OF LIVE TEACHERS. How does this translate into reality? Having seen no empirical studies of health teachers in action, I shall have to suggest some impressions . . . and if these diverge from those of others, then there may be a basis for more systematic study. In general, teachers in the elementary grades are most oriented to the learning process, and those at the college and university levels are most oriented to the content of the field. Secondary teachers are rather in-between, but probably have a bit more orientation toward the college level than toward the elementary level.

Some teachers possess minds that truly generate ideas and can genuinely communicate ideas and concepts to learners. The examples selected or developed and the particular words and phrases chosen by them do communicate with many learners. These are very special people. Some writers fit this description also; their written words communicate decidedly better than most published material. It probably is true that considerably more teachers and writers consider themselves to be in this category than truly belong there. In Hindu tradition, the genuine, enlightened guru never designates himself as such, but merely responds as seekers after wisdom acknowledge him and seek him out. The truly enlightened one never has to tell another; if it is real, it shines forth. This probably applies to the unique teacher also. She/he possesses wisdom in relation to health, and there is no direct way to attain this condition of wisdom or to increase it. It just happens with a few, and fortunate are those learners who have some contact with them.

Some well-informed teachers, probably more likely in the elementary and lower secondary grades, can organize learning situations for real interaction and genuine active learning. They personally have developed important health concepts, but they possess the patience and the insight to let students develop comparable ones on their own, at their own rates. This teaching ability can be increased with practice and with desire, and can be improved through in-service experiences and interaction with creative colleagues. The ability, however, needs to be combined with the aforementioned patience and perception so that students really do learn more effectively under this strategy. To be this kind of facilitator of learning requires no special ability akin to that of the previously described ideal idealist. It does require a pronounced faith in students and their ability and desire to learn, if motivated and guided . . . and it does require efficacious learning activities. The art of feeling just what is the right type of activity, when, and for how long is some part gift and some part persistent work.

Probably most teachers, at all levels, give assignments, pass on information, administer tests, and decided how achievements translate into grades. This is a set of basic functions, easier to perform than either of the other styles, and, from an administrative standpoint, the simplest to replace, temporarily or permanently.

SOME RECOLLECTIONS. Each of these represents assumptions about the reality of learning. If all learners were fundamentally alike, then one might be true and the others false. But the counter hypothesis I shall offer is that there are enough different types of learners to give each style a demonstrable validity.

"I'll always remember Mr. Malcolm . . . he just had a special way of making health interesting. Things I had learned before now made sense after he explained them . . . there aren't very many teachers like Mr. Malcolm."

"Remember Ms. Hardaway? Her lectures were really well organized and they coordinated so well with the text and the outside reading that you really learned a lot in her class. She had a real thing about the need for discipline in learning, and when you kept up in her class, it really did discipline your mind . . . and you learned."

"Do I remember my health class? I sure do. I'm not sure who the teacher was, but she sure did organize some interesting activities. I learned more about people, how they think, and the differences in values that are behind healthy and unhealthy behavior than in any other class. And I really didn't realize all of the benefits at the time. But as time goes on, I keep realizing what I'm learning now is something that began in the health class. What was that teacher's name?

WHAT WE EXPERIENCE. We learn from what we experience. Perhaps it is true that everything we experience becomes part of us or is learned, some in the conscious and the rest in the unconscious. If it is true, it has tremendous implications, but, for this discussion, let us focus on the conscious. We learn from experience, and the more we focus attention on the experience, the more predictable the learning will be. Conditioning processes reward the concentration on the right elements of the experiences and ignore other responses. The desires for inner satisfaction, recognition, and reward urge the learner to repeat those behaviors that bring the benefits. The learning experience that results in conscious inner satisfaction is likely to be both a remembered and a repeated one. The less distracting the experience, the more likely that learning takes place. However, there is no way that one person can make another person—or a class of persons—learn.

So, a single example of clear-cut, uncluttered learning experience . . .

"For the rest of the hour, I want all of you to read and study pages 89-99. There will be no talking, no other work, and no moving around the room." This has the advantage of outwardly forcing attention on one source of stimulation and allowing a minimum of distracting influences, but has the disadvantage of providing only one stimulus. If the words and ideas on page 89 do nothing to excite Sharon's mind, it moves away to choices of clothes, whom she likes and whom she doesn't, what her mother meant by that last remark this morning. There are going to be no other stimuli to bring her back to the book and get her on to pages 90, 91, and through 99.

Those who are intrinsically interested in the content and those who have self-discipline to bring themselves back from mind-wanderings (for whatever number of reasons) will learn from this type of teaching-learning strategy. Those without these requisites will learn less.

On the other hand, an example of an active, cluttered learning experience . . .

"Move into small groups as they are set up on the overhead projector, select a leader and a recorder, select a proposition from those on the board and then pool all the information you have from the group on this proposition. Decide where and how you will get more information and proceed. By Thursday at this time, each group should be ready to dramatize some of the implications of its chosen proposition before the class. If you have questions, I shall be available to help. Otherwise, get to work."

The latter learning experience has the advantage of containing many stimuli, so that when any individual's attention wanders, there are many ways to bring it back. Further, since the group has to accomplish the task, there are pressures to help one another. Peers will urge Sharon's wandering attention back to the task. There also are different skills required so that the person who does not read well, for instance, still may contribute something and learn something. This example of a learning experience has the disadvantage of having built into it myriad distractions. The group may or may not be personally compatible, choosing a leader may be distracting from the task, and the major learning for Sharon in the whole three days may be what a dingbat Jerry is.

BUT ONE FITS U.S. CULTURE BETTER. Each strategy has certain pros and cons. Perhaps a choice of one general direction or the other is a rather free one. Perhaps not. If students of today were growing up in a consistent, stable culture where youngsters were to be seen and not heard—where adults clearly held dominance over children and youth—then a strategy of merely giving an assignment or telling a class what they should know would be quite appropriate. If general expectations about life within the culture were not high, meaning that jobs, marriages, meals, etc., were expected to be rather dull, hum-drum, uninteresting, and non-provocative, then educational experiences of dull, repetitive assignments directed by an authoritative adult would be appropriate. Under these conditions, those who could, would learn, and those who couldn't, would simply drop out and do one of the many things in life that required no special schooling.

But present American culture is brimming over with stimuli of various kinds, and people are urged, from childhood, to respond to the most satisfying. Jobs, meals, marriages, etc., are supposed to be personally satisfying and fulfilling, and there's very little credence given to the "life is supposed to be hard" philosophy. For learners who are attentive, participating members of this culture, then, learning activities that seem interesting and promise some possibility of enjoyment are more likely to attract and hold attention. And where attention is, there is learning more likely.

In a culture where an individual's failure to learn was his or her own loss only, Mr. Dillard's statement that "I put it out for them to learn . . . if they haven't the gumption to take the opportunity, they'll just be sorry" was probably fitting. But in our culture, the taxpayers who did learn are going to have to pay for those who didn't. The cost of people's choosing to live in unhealthy ways will be large enough. It seems imperative that we try, with some of the zeal and skill of those trying to sell products, to reduce the cost of people's living unhealthfully *out of ignorance*. An ecological slogan from an earlier chapter was:

Everything is connected to everything else.

There is a monetary and social cost to not making efforts to get all students to learn as much as possible.

DIFFERENT SENSES. Finally, we have five basic senses, and we learn through all of them . . . and all of them can help hinder learning. Individuals differ in how much they can learn from listening and reading. Individuals differ in how well they can grasp principles without examples. Varied approaches to learning seem to embody the democratic notion that no one way of learning is necessarily superior to others.

EXAMPLES. Those who tire of academic musings without examples may have quit reading some time back. At any rate, here are some examples of teaching-learning strategies in health, described by a teacher or learning director, with a short pro and con argument for each. In general, the order represents a continuum from the most passive for a class to the most active.

1. *Lecture.* "I lectured to the class on the dynamics of population. I gathered the information from many sources to which most of them would not have had access. It was a straight lecture and it took the whole period. Their notes will be better than any single book they could read."

   Pro. The teacher who is a good scholar in any of the sub-fields of health may be able to synthesize facts and ideas in a unique and useful way, and may be able to present them in a clear, compelling, interesting fashion. This saves learners time, and if their motivations are high, the lecture is a very effective method.

Con. Each chapter in a text or other reference book is a synthesis by a scholar or group of scholars, generally more academically competent and talented in use of words than many teachers, so the lecture may be just a duplication. It is essentially passive for the learner and involves learning by hearing. Those who are not highly motivated may have difficulty following the systematic presentation.

2. *Lecture/Demonstration.* "The lecture I gave today was illustrated. I wrote on the board and showed two pictures and several graphs. It was a good, systematic presentation on causes and numbers of accidents. It would have been harder to grasp without the presentations."

Pro. The illustrated lecture has the same advantages as the straight lecture with the additional offering of some relevant stimuli for the eye, an additional sense. When two senses are involved, there is more chance of learning. If the lecture includes some story-telling (using the description of some human experience, actual or made-up, serious or funny, as an illustration), it is more apt to hold listeners' interest.

Con. Essentially the same disadvantages—largely passive. If the pictures, graphs and illustrations are not large enough to be seen by all, they become a frustrating distraction rather than a helpful addition.

3. *Films.* "I used a film in class today. It was on venereal disease, and it certainly did a better job than I could of covering both the scientific and human aspects of these conditions. It was 38 minutes long, and, with the time it took to get started and the film breaking once, it took the whole period. There was no time for discussion."

Pro. The film has all the advantages of the lecture and, in addition, can offer a variety of speakers, demonstrations and graphic illustrations. A film can create a mood, can tell a story, and can affect the emotions. It, along with a television program seen in class, the filmstrip and slides, presents experiences for the eyes and ears of listeners to behold that they might never encounter otherwise.

Con. Though a good film (or strip or set of slides) can stimulate the mind and the emotions, it is typically a physically passive, sitting experience. For youngsters raised on exciting television fare, some educational films may seem dull . . . and some are. If there is no time for discussion afterward, some students may leave with some misconceptions about the topic. These may be harder to change at a later time than when the viewing is immediately past and perceptions can be checked with those of the teacher and other screen-watchers.

4. *Multiple Demonstrations.* "I just had a great class! It was my anti-smoking lesson in which I used a short film, models of lungs (one healthy, one of a heavy smoker, and one really diseased), smoking Sam, and a demonstration of blowing cigarette smoke into a clean white handkerchief. There was time for a little discussion at the end, but not much . . . that's a lot to do in one class period. The kids seemed really interested."

Pro. The variety of visual and auditory stimuli can do much to capture and keep attention. To demonstrate something, to have a model of what is being talked about . . . each has the potential for making something clear that otherwise would just have been words. If some students can be involved in demonstrations, and if they can examine models up close, the chances for attention—and learning—increase.

Con. Still a physically passive, watching-listening experience for most. Live demonstrations may not show what they are supposed to. Models may create false impressions. Without discussion and follow-up, you can never be sure what students have taken away from such a well-planned, many-stimuli presentation.

5. *Guest Speaker.* "I had a guest speaker in class today. She used several transparencies, some professionally prepared and some she had done herself. She essentially lectured, but allowed time for questions and answers at the end. She was good, but I think if I invite her again, I'll interview her in front of the class."

Pro. A guest speaker introduces a different voice, personality and set of experiences into the class setting . . . and presumably she/he has some particular expertise to share. Transparencies present large visual images that supplement a lecture and can be projected without dimming lights or pulling blinds and without the speaker changing positions. The visuals themselves can be informational, symbolic, situational, provocative, or combinations thereof. Interviewing a guest helps the teacher keep control. This method can almost assure that the speaker will deal with the issues relevant to the class and that the speaker doesn't get sidetracked on some side issues or experience.

Con. A guest speaker is another passive, listening experience for youngsters, She/he may have expertise, but may not communicate well with youngsters. She/he may or may not stick to the topic. Some transparencies may be of poor quality, particularly home-made ones. The interview may turn into a way for the teacher to "ride his/her own hobby horse." Students then seem to hear a replay of the teacher rather than a different, fresh approach.

6. *Panel-Debate.* "I can't decide whether to have the kids finish up this unit on mood modifying substances with a debate or just a panel. Which would you do?"

Pro. A debate usually points at some specific issues while a panel can be more wide-ranging. A debate, because it tends to be more competitive, may be more lively. Each involves activity for those selected to debate or panel, and, if organized appropriately, can involve all class members in preparation. Both give students a chance to hear student opinions and interpretations.

Con. A debate for which the participants have prepared well can leave one side (perhaps even both) feeling extreme about some issue in which the extreme is not a healthy attitude. For the non-participants, the debate or the panel is an essentially passive experience. It can also be a negative one if the chosen speakers are not liked by some students. Particularly in a debate, participants may present untruths or interpret facts in distorted ways. A teacher must decide, at that point, to correct the point and probably spoil the debate, or she can wait and hope to make the correction at a more appropriate time.

7. *Sociodrama-Skit.* "We started the class off today with a series of short sociodramas—a clinic physician dealing with a series of different kids with venereal disease. We then spent the rest of the hour discussing the difference in reactions and in correcting and reinforcing the factual statements made. It kept the class' interest and gave us a referent to go back to throughout the whole hour. Another class decided to have a skit instead, and one group presented venereal disease in a conversation between a gonococcus and a spirochete inside a boy's body. That was a provocative start to a class, I'll tell you!"

Pro. A sociodrama or a skit is an opportunity to create a living, human flavor in a topic. The interaction in a sociodrama is unplanned, so the spontaneous responses can be valuable indicators of attitudes and present understandings. A skit is planned and rehearsed, so that what is presented is the distillation of all that could have been. Both are active experiences for the participants and may be enjoyable, as well as thought-provoking, for the rest of the class.

Con. Any classroom dramatization runs the risk of being a fiasco. It may be dull and repetitive. It may emphasize unimportant points or get away from the central topic entirely. A skit may be worse than a sociodrama because there is planned interchange, but insufficient rehearsal may leave one or more actors unprepared and unpredictable, which certainly threatens the potential for being a useful classroom experience.

8. *Discussion.* "We have lots of class discussion in the health classes. Some of it comes after a lecture or a film, some of it could be called problem-solving, some deals with a particular human case or group in a situation. Sometimes the whole class is involved together, but at least once a week we do something with small group discussions."

Pro. Class discussion is a basic way in which a learner tries out what she/he knows, finds out what she/he doesn't, and has what she/he believes to be truth reinforced and corrected. Discussion can deal just with facts and abstractions or with human life situations. Both have merit in health education. In the total class discussion the teacher is directly involved most of the time, can hear all that the students say, and can offer the authoritative word when such is needed. In a small group discussion, more students have a chance to speak and, because the teacher is not directly involved, some things may be said that would be otherwise inhibited.

Con. Class discussion often involves an exercise in verbal gymnastics between the teacher and several verbal students or, if the teacher is so inclined, an opportunity for a series of lecturettes, planned or spontaneous. A teacher may ask a question, receive an inadequate answer, and then proceed to answer her/his own question . . . and then comment that "we had a good discussion in my last hour class today." Small group discussions can be a sharing of ignorance . . . or an opportunity for one or more students to dominate with their opinions, worthy or unworthy. The fact that students seem to enjoy discussion does not mean it necessarily increases learning. It may . . . or it may not . . . or may set desired learning backward by teaching and reinforcing some inaccurate views.

9. *Current Events.* "We start each Monday with an analysis of current events relating to the topic we're on . . . sometimes to health in general. This includes analysis of any radio or tele-

vision programs, public service announcements, or whatever needs analyzing. Some Mondays there isn't much going on, but typically the class period is over before we've analyzed everything that has been offered as current."

Pro. This kind of activity helps make students aware that what they are learning in health is related to current happenings . . . and that what is learned in a classroom has utility and is related to the outside world—the community beyond the classroom. It encourages reading of newspapers and news magazines and a listening-viewing frame of reference geared to more than entertainment.

Con. Current events can involve anything that is happening at the moment, much of which is of no lasting importance. Interest may be aroused, attention given, and opinions formed and reformed about some happening that is never verified, replicated, or even remembered by health-related professionals. With limited time for classroom learning, this activity may be worth the time it takes.

10. *Survey.* "My children did a survey, in which each child checked his or her own home, garage, and yards for hazards."
    Pro. This survey is a way of relating the home or larger community to the concern being studied in the classroom. It is an active learning experience for everyone who participates, one that can help sharpen abilities to observe according to some criteria.

    Con. The purposes and/or the content of a survey may be misunderstood by some of the student surveyors . . . and certainly by some of those being surveyed or other people in the community. Such misunderstandings may cause more trouble for the teacher or the school than what can be learned is worth. Surveys (such as the one described) may serve to highlight the differences between the various students' homes that have ramifications beyond mere objective safety. Some learning about social class and economic differences can be painful, though important.

11. *Creative Writing.* "After discussing the story, in diary form, of a boy's developing undesirable patterns of eating, I had the students write a story, play, poem, or any other creative form. This assignment was to be about a person their age, but of the opposite sex, developing new food likes for various reasons. I'm reading them now, and some of these kids are very creative!"
    Pro. To the extent that health education is based on past experiences of others, it can be factual; to the extent that it

deals with predicting the future, it can be creative. Creativity in thinking opens the mind to new possibilities in thinking . . . and behaving. Creative writing is tangible evidence of creative thinking. It can show ways a student thinks that are not revealed on tests or by more standard assignments. A teacher may save and use a creative story as a teaching instrument for subsequent class.

Con. Some youngsters have little creative ability, and a creative writing assignment can be rather frustrating. For others the creative experience may be seductive; they get carried away with the writing and the style and lose the point or purpose for the assignment. Some students may be more creative than the teacher, and the teacher cannot fairly evaluate what they produce.

12. *Games.* "My ninth-grade class decided that learning about food selection and eating patterns and nutrition was usually pretty dull . . . and it needn't be. So we set up a week's workshop to develop games to teach this important health-related area at the sixth-grade level. After the games were developed and built, we had two days of demonstrating and playing them."

Pro. To play a game you have to know something (whatever the game is about). Because most games are somehow competitive, motives to learn are almost inherent. The game can be fun and exciting . . . and still be educational. Devising, building, and playing a game involves almost maximum activity on the part of learners in the workshop setting.

Con. The danger, as in other creative activities, is that the game is excellent and exciting, but learning can be minimal. All of this creation, development and playing takes time, which might be better spent on activities with more predictable learning outcome.

13. *Field Trip.* "We went on a field trip to the sewage treatment plant. It was well-conducted, and the kids got to see how the whole process works—from the dirty water coming in to the clean, pure water going out."

Pro. A book or a lecture or even a picture can describe and portray something like a sewage treatment plant, but, for many youngsters, it remains a shadowy abstraction. A visit to the plant actually brings it into the concrete. With a good guide, who can speak in terms the class group can understand, the trip can be an active, satisfying learning experience.

Con. Only parts of anything can be seen, and these may not be very important. When something is explained, typically part of the class cannot hear or see. Disciplinary problems may detract from actual learning; there are always some who are not interested in whatever it is and take advantage of relative freedom. Field trips have to be scheduled well in advance. When a trip is held, it may not be appropriate, the weather may be inappropriate, or what has to be seen is not available.

A CONTINUUM. There are, of course, many other methods and techniques to induce learning. Even with combinations, no one could claim that thirteen descriptions represent the universe. However, adding others would not change the basic generalizations to which these thirteen analyses point.

Teaching-Learning Strategies Are Represented on a
Continuum,
the Poles of Which Are

Teacher as   Student as
Teacher   Learner

Teachers utilizing strategies to the left of center have, as their dominant thoughts,

". . . My responsibility as a teacher is to see that the students learn the right things . . . and to see that they don't learn the wrong things. . . . I know the subject matter well, and it seems a waste of time not to have the students take full advantage of this. . . . You have to create and maintain an atmosphere for learning in the classroom, and in order to do this the teacher must be the authority figure at all times. . . . There just isn't enough time to use some of those student participation methods. . . . The content becomes greater each year, and it is my responsibility to see that youngsters learn as much of it as possible. . . . I have to use the most efficient methods. . . ."

Teachers choosing more approaches from the right side would have, as their chief guiding thoughts,

". . . My responsibility as a teacher is primarily as a facilitator of learning . . . as well as a provider of information . . . it is to see that the youngsters learn how to learn and to know that they know a variety of ways to learn. . . . There probably are a few things that everyone should learn and know are right. . . . With all health topics or concepts, there is more than can be learned. . . . I'd rather a student learn something that seems valuable to him/her than simply not learn something that I thought was important. . . . The atmosphere to create is one of mutual learning . . . I am a learner, too, and can learn things from students. . . . If students ask me for information they want and need, this is also a way to learn; seeking authority is applicable beyond the classroom, while lecturing them before they need to know tends not to be.

. . . I don't know any ways to make learning more effective given the heterogeneous group of students I have in each class. . . ."

And so it goes. . . . Some teachers will be truly eclectic, and their teaching-learning direction will display a comfortably, honest balance of approaches from all over the continuum:

Monday:	Lecture
Tuesday:	Small group discussion
Wednesday:	Full period film
Thursday:	Panel discussion
Friday:	Choice of objective test or creative writing project

Others, however, will have some of the following difficulties:

- Believing in strategies on the right of the continuum, but having more tangible success and feeling of accomplishment with the ones on the left

- Feeling, as a young idealistic teacher, that approaches from the right of the continuum are best, but being coerced by supervising teachers and departmental policies to use more from the left side of the continuum

- Believing, idealistically, in strategies on the right continuum but having little natural ability and confidence in trying them; without trying, there is no success and without success there is no development of ability and confidence

- Believing in the strategies on the left continuum, but being coerced by younger, eager colleagues and by nondocile students to try some approaches that one does not really believe in

- Believing in strategies from the right continuum, but having knowledge that "I learned satisfactorily by left-end strategies" and reverting to teaching as one was taught.

NO SINGLE BEST ONE. A recurring theme in this volume is that no teaching-learning approach is best for everyone, and there is also probably none from which someone does not learn. Each teacher must decide for her/himself what strategies to use. Whatever one does for a period of time can have some rewards and become comfortable.

REALIZING SOME OBJECTIVES. Another view of teaching-learning strategies comes from suggesting several ways in which a particular semi-behavioral objective could be realized. Let's look at these also in terms of maturity-age levels.

Level I (Kindergarten, grades, 1, 2, and 3)
Identifies procedures that help protect personal well-being and that of others

"After talking about protecting health, our teacher read us a story and we raised our hands every time somebody did something good for his or her health . . . or for somebody else's."

"For about the last two weeks, we've been making a list of things people do to keep healthy and another of things that aren't good for you. The lists are on our bulletin board so that we can read them and add to them if we think of more."

"Our teacher printed each thing on both lists [see above] on a card. Now we play a game, where someone comes up, draws a card from the pile, reads the 'procedure' (the teacher calls it) and puts it in the 'helpful' or 'harmful' pile. If we think it is a wrong choice, we can say so."

Describes all that happens when a person is sick

"Each of us had to think of a time when we were sick and then all that happened during and because of that illness . . . the consequences, the teacher called them. Then some of us got to tell ours out loud and the teacher recorded them so we could hear them again."

"Each of us read a story about a brother and sister being sick and then three people got to come up and tell the story about all the things that happened because they were sick. Then we got to make up some other things that could have happened instead . . . or after the story ended."

Level II (grades 4, 5, and 6)

Explains how and why problems may result from
an unbalanced diet and from a certain lack of foods

"We've been studying this and now we've made up two sets of cards—one describing problems and the other describing particular unbalanced diets and lack of certain foods. We sit in a circle and one person draws a card and reads it aloud, and then gives it to someone else who has to explain aloud either how or why the problem happened."

"Each of us had to write four letters to four persons with health problems described on a printed sheet; the letters had to explain how and why the problem occurred and what they should do to their diet to correct them."

Compare individual growth status with
information contained in growth charts

"Each of us was weighed and measured at the beginning of the year. Each of us who was in the school last year had the information from last year, too. Now, near the end of the year, we got weighed and measured again and each of us gets to see how our growth compares with a growth chart on the bulletin board."

"Each of us makes up a person who weighed so much and was so tall last year and this year. Then we exchange with someone so that they can compare the growth of my made-up person with the chart. Then we write about these made-up persons."

*Illustrates relationships between accidents
and human behavior*

"We gathered some pictures of accidents. Each person has a picture and three half-sheets of blank paper. We make up a story about how the accident happened. We pass the papers around so everyone writes on three. Then we pass them around and read the different stories people made up. A committee decides the five best ones for posting on the bulletin board."

"We made up a list of how people act—you know, like over-sleeping in the morning, etc. Two of the class members read them on a casette tape. Now we turn on the tape and someone has to give an example of how the way people act might cause accidents."

Level III (grades 7, 8, and 9)

Analyzes the qualifications for various health careers

"Through library research and interviews, our class developed a set of qualifications for fifteen different careers related to health. Now each person is assigned one and can choose two others . . . we have to write an analysis of each, telling what kinds of people would do well in the career. Then we compare our analyses with at least two others who have analyzed the same one."

"We had a health career day with about twelve different speakers. We taped what they said, and now we listen to the tapes and have a panel analyze the qualifications for each—what they are, how they might change, who could meet them, etc."

*Evaluates those social forces and emotional factors
that encourage and discourage good dental care*

"From our combined experience, our class made up two lists of social forces and emotional factors that encourage and that discourage dental care. Then we had six teams that interviewed two dentists, two dental hygienists, and two dental receptionists to see which of them were felt to be the most important. Each report was made, and we made up a composite report of their evaluations. Each could then compare it with his own judgment."

"We had a debate in class, with one side arguing that social and emotional factors that encourage good dental care are stronger, and the other arguing that those that discourage good dental care are stronger. Each person had to cast a ballot indicating his judgment as to which side won—and why."

Level IV (grades 10, 11, and 12)

*Formulates hypotheses on what it would be like
if there were no differences among individuals*

"We worked in groups of three, and each group formulated a description of the universal person—everyone alive would fit this description. We then passed these around to see how they were alike and how they were different. Then each group had to write on two, formulating hypotheses as to what a culture of these people would be like. These eventually were typed up and put in our classroom library. It kind of stretches your mind to read it."

"We formulated our universal person like the other class did, but then we each had to interview three people not in the class and then, as a group, we had to put these hypotheses of what life would be like together."

Integrates data into an effective plan for
the solution of a family life problem

"We read a bunch of 'Dear Abby' columns and then by written vote decided on six family life problems to solve. Each person signed up for one, and then had to find published data to back up every suggested part of the plan."

"We worked backwards. We gathered, as a class, a lot of data on family life problems. Then we put the data together in different forms and tried to predict what problems these might help solve."

Translates knowledge about the effects of various
mood and behavior modifiers into predictions about the
behavior of those who use them under different circumstances

"For about a month we, as a class, collected news stories of different kinds of behavior in different circumstances, some of which involved mood modifiers and some not. Then on a particular day we worked in pairs of students, and each pair was given a news item. We had to research the behavior and match it with the effects of some modifiers. Then the next day, as many as possible gave their interpretations, translating the knowledge about effects into a prediction about cause of the behavior described."

"Our teacher, who has had some special training in education about alcohol and drugs, gave a really great lecture in which he translated facts about effects of different substances into predictions about how different people would react under different circumstances. It certainly helped us to think about the whole drug issue."

IN SUMMARY.

- The two ends of a continuum of teaching-learning strategies are: emphasis on the teacher as (1) purveyor of knowledge and (2) organizer of learning experiences and facilitator of learning.
- Some teachers can be comfortably and effectively eclectic in strategies, but there are forces pulling teachers in both directions so some are not comfortable with their teaching style.

- Learning comes from the learner focusing attention; different activities accomplish this differently; an activity is effective for those who respond with focused attention.
- There are pros and cons to every learning activity.
- There always are several ways for a class to accomplish an objective.
- This culture is one that can ill afford learning failures; there are fewer and fewer functional roles for the uneducated.

Chapter XIII

Materials and Resources

"My students are using a variety of books, magazines, and journals from the library in addition to those available in our classrooms; these give them a much wider view of any health issue than just a textbook."

"My students went to the library to use a wider range of materials; many of the books were out or otherwise not available, some magazines and journals were missing and others had the desired article cut out. Some of the important ones were away being bound. It was a frustrating, and not very rewarding, experience. I'm glad we have the textbook."

"I used a film as the culminating learning experience for this unit, and it was excellent. It pictured many of the issues we had considered in the abstract, and it reinforced the feeling that I had tried to encourage. The discussion afterward indicated it was really appreciated."

"The film I really wanted to culminate the unit was not available until a week after the unit was over. I ordered another film, it was confirmed, but there was a holiday the day before, the mail was late, and it arrived two days after it was supposed to. It's probably just as well . . . the last time I used a film, it broke in one dramatic spot and the bulb burned out in another."

"I've had students use the prepared visual transparencies that we have available in group presentations they make to the class. These make the presentations more interesting and better learning experiences. The students learn a great deal in going through the sets of visuals, selecting ones that are most appropriate."

"I've encouraged students to use the prepared visual transparencies that we have available in group presentations to the class. After one year the librarian says five have been damaged so that they are unusable, and seven are missing, lost or stolen. I hate to penalize the majority for what a minority does, but we have no money to replace these. At this rate, there will be none left for teacher use in a few years. So, no more student use."

These antithetical conversations are intended to represent two truths about supplemental resource materials for learning in health:

1. A variety of high quality instructional materials are available to add feeling, informational and experience dimensions to classroom learning experiences.

2. These materials typically have to be shared, and therefore the availability of just what is desired is dependent on many other people, some of whom have less than desired responsibility. These add up to the generalization that resource materials can be extremely enriching and/or a source of great frustration. Teachers who use them find ways to minimize these frustrations or simply have personalities that can tolerate the failures with the successes. Teachers who do not have such tolerance often protect themselves from this frustration by developing other teaching strategies or profess to believe that the time spent arranging for efficient use could be better used in other forms of learning direction.

CHOICES AND DECISIONS. Some resource materials cost a school or district money, and someone—or some group—must be continually deciding how much to allocate for all such materials. Because this is rarely enough to cover all things from which learners might benefit— how much to spend for what? to buy or to rent? transparencies vs. films? another movie projector or a not presently available slide projector? money for field trips or another television set? The choices are numerous and complex. Technology produces new types and styles of hardware, and publishers multiply the types and varieties of software. Patent laws have lost some effectiveness because by the time a suit against a competing company for violating a patent comes to court, the machine in question is likely to have been superseded by a new model.

What is good quality and worth the purchase or rental price is a question for continual judgment. In late 1972, the National Coordinating Council on Drug Education [1] released a report that judged only 34 audio-visual aids—16 percent of the 220 reviewed—to be "scientifically accurate and conceptually sound." The major generalization was offered that the drug abuse films available today are doing more harm than good. This was the Council's considered corporate judgment, but the fact remains that many of the films and other materials that flunked were made by recognized film-makers, many with medical and educational advisors. If the decision-maker in an audio-visual department is confronted with this report and a request from four health teachers for a film not approved, what does he do? How much time can he take to decide how to decide? Oh, well. Whatever the complexities, resource materials are an important part of the curriculum and teaching-learning strategies of most health teachers.

---

[1] "Drug Council Finds 16% of Drug Abuse Films 'Scientifically Acceptable,'" *Drugs and Drug Abuse Education Newsletter.* Washington, D.C.: Scope Publications, December 1972. pp. 4, 5.

AUDIO-VISUAL MATERIALS are those that students can hear and/or see and usually refer to other than texts or other standard-type books. Audio-visual materials should rarely be considered ends in themselves. Their value is in helping to make learning more effective.

Some guidelines for the use of these instructional materials may be summarized as follows:

1. All audio-visual materials are a means of helping to achieve educational objectives. The selection of these materials should be guided by what is to be taught and what the desired outcomes are.

2. Each aid has its advantages and its limitations. For any specific situation, the teacher has to select the learning aid or combination of aids that will be most helpful to the learners. With guidance, learners may also develop judgment in selection.

3. Audio-visual materials are not merely substitutes for other instructional techniques. They are an integral part of teaching, and can serve only to reinforce and supplement other forms of instruction.

4. The mere exposure to audio-visual materials will not assure learning that is meaningful. Careful planning and preparation and follow-up are necessary if any kind of teaching is to serve as a channel for enriched learning experiences.

5. The skillful use of audio-visual materials encourages the pupil to assume responsibility for his own learning by helping him to organize, interpret, integrate, and apply what is being taught. These features guide the learner into an active role, rather than a passive one.

EDUCATIONAL VALUES. Research in the use of audio-visual materials offers assurance that certain values can be attributed to the use of these materials if the proper guidelines for their use are observed, Hoban, Finn, and Dale [2] conclude that audio-visual materials, when correctly used in teaching, can accomplish the following:

1. Supply a concrete basis for conceptual thinking and reduce meaningless word responses of pupils

2. Engender a high degree of interest in pupils

3. Make learning more permanent

4. Offer a reality of experience that stimulates pupil self-activity

5. Develop a continuity of thought. (This is especially true of motion pictures.)

---

[2] Hoban, Charles F., Finn, James, and Dale, Edgar, "Audiovisual Materials," *Encyclopedia of Educational Research.* New York: MacMillan, 1950. pg. 84.

6. Contribute to growth of meaning and to vocabulary development

7. Provide experiences not easily obtained through other materials and contribute to the efficiency, depth and variety of learning

DEMONSTRATIONS. The teacher may use a demonstration, or visualized explanation, to show how something operates, how it is done, or to show cause-effect relationships. In the demonstration, she draws on many other teaching materials that are available to illustrate a given concept. A step-by-step procedure for applying artificial ventilation, a comparison of pulse count at rest and following varying degrees of activity, clarification of the parts and functions of the human ear with a cutaway model, a chronological explanation of the menstrual cycle with a chart or model, an experiment to show the conditions under which disease-producing organisms thrive—all these are examples of demonstrations.

The teacher may tell a class how something is constructed or how it functions. To add reality, she/he illustrates her/his explanation with a demonstration. Whenever appropriate and practical, she/he allows the pupils to perform the demonstration themselves. This opportunity for doing on the part of the class is especially desirable in health and safety education where the learning of a skill or pattern of behavior is a primary goal. First aid and driver education are almost wholly dependent on individual practice by the pupils following the teacher's demonstration, if learning is to be reinforced and lasting.

The successful demonstration emerges from an admixture of simple design, clarity of explanation, and advanced preparation of materials to be used. In addition, the teacher needs to be thoroughly familiar with the subject, to communicate well during the demonstration, and to be cognizant of the salient points in the demonstration. It is necessary, of course, that the demonstration be visible to all pupils. The quality of the questions and the kinds of class comments during the demonstration and following it are pretty good barometers of how much real learning is taking place.

EXHIBITS. When time and distance present limitations to the widening of educational horizons, the teacher considers ways of providing the learner with a replica of the real situation or environment. Exhibits, which rely on arrangements of objects, models, specimens, or mock-ups (scale models), are planned to convey a specific message to the viewer.

When an object or specimen of the real thing is not available, or is impractical for display purposes, a three-dimensional likeness or model, scaled up or down, can be constructed or obtained from commercial sources. Such representations are best when authentic, but sometimes a simplified version is necessary. In these instances, the teacher points out to the class the omission of certain parts of the original, so that inaccurate impressions will not be formed.

The cutaway model has advantages as a learning aid in that it enables pupils to view the interior structure or workability of some specific organ that is not outwardly visible. For example, a model of the eye or ear, with removable parts, lends itself to examination and broader understanding of the importance of each part in the total functioning of the organ.

The diorama is a three-dimensional representation of a scene with the objects and models positioned in proper perspective within a replica of their natural environment. In a unit of study devoted to community health, for example, there are many phases of this topic that lend themselves to presentation through the use of the diorama. A comprehension of the potential hazards that confront a driver on the highway and in congested traffic centers can be gained readily from a realistic arrangement in a diorama. The instructional value of the diorama in health education, when pupil-made, has two benefits: the study of the finished scene and the construction process. In the construction process, many decisions about truth, perspective, appropriateness, etc., must be made, which are learning opportunities.

There are many things that contribute to the efficacy of an exhibit. Motion, viewer participation, accuracy of detail, location of the exhibit, brevity and clarity of captions, illuminations, and color are points to be considered. Although the exhibit is often placed within the school environment, real advantages may accrue by locating the exhibit in a community setting to instruct citizens and to help them appreciate the civic-minded concern of pupils for health problems.

The educational health museum, a fine resource in some communities, enriches school curricula. Pupil observation in the museum needs adequate time and expert guidance. A hurried and unorganized museum tour can lead to confusion and misunderstanding. The exhibits in a legitimate health museum are authentic, attractive, and dynamic, and they cover a wide range of topics in personal, family and community health. Some of the exhibit materials are available for loan to schools. The health museums provide additional services, such as the orientation of teachers for the optimal use of museum facilities, preparation of resource materials, lectures and group discussions.

FIELD TRIPS. A field trip is a unique, moving experience in which the classroom is extended into the community. It may be a planned visit to some place within the school or its environs, or a journey to some point within the community. The latter is particularly significant for the contribution it can make to narrowing the gap between school experiences and community life. More extensive field trips may require traveling a considerable distance and may last a period of several days.

Some school systems issue a guidebook that has been developed for teachers on the basis of past experiences with field trips. The teacher will find this item a valuable reference. It typically lists the available resources in each community, school regulations and suggested procedures for planning the field experience. Usually the guide also classifies the trips that are suitable for various age groups, and helps to eliminate duplication of trips students have taken at earlier grade levels.

In most communities, there are numerous opportunities that can be assessed for their potential contribution to health and safety education. Visits might be made to laboratories food processing plants, produce markets, water purification plants, sewage disposal plants, governmental agencies, traffic centers, pharmaceutical firms, industrial establishments, research centers, museums, and clinics and hospitals during open house or at other appropriate times. The maturity level and intellectual background of the pupils will govern the type of visit to be made. Although the large metropolitan areas are richer in the resources they have to offer, some studies suggest that school systems located in smaller communities often utilize the available resources to a greater extent. Obviously, the complexity of the administrative arrangements, particularly time, safety, and transportation, serves as an obstacle to more frequent field trips. However, once the values of field trips are recognized, a teacher can find ways to overcome such obstacles. For example, when the field trips are administratively difficult, small groups or individuals may make the excursion and then report to the class, serving as a fair substitute.

The field trip is often used as a motivating device, and in this sense, it serves as a good introduction to a unit of study. It may be planned during the unit to enhance the learning and clarify some specific segment of a unit. Or it may be selected as the procedure that will serve best at the termination of a unit to bring the learning experience to an understandable focus.

Essentially, the same educational principles that underlie the use of other teaching aids apply to the field trip as a learning activity. It is imperative that the reason for the field trip be clear to both the teacher and the pupils, because what is learned through the experience depends largely on the purpose and planning agreed on at the outset.

When a field trip is called successful, the need for the trip probably arose as a natural outgrowth of classroom study, and students developed an awareness of the purposes and values of their trip. The use of other teaching materials during the stages of preparation helped to enhance the value of the experience. Pupils and teacher shared in formulating the observations they hoped to make and the questions they wanted to have answered. Since a guide is usually assigned by the host group, he/

she needs advance notice of the class' expectations, so that the visitors and personnel at the community resource are in accord with each other's purpose.

Preparations for a field trip prior to the community visit are perhaps more extensive and detailed than those for use of most other teaching procedures. Often in this learning situation, an entire class goes to the scene of the learning activity rather than bringing the learning aid into the classroom. This type of field trip requires meticulous attention to administrative details, transportation, arrangements with the community resources to be visited, parental permission, appropriate clothing, standards of behavior, time allotment, changes in class schedule, safety factors, and adequate supervision. However, when carefully planned and conducted, a field trip can:

1. Encourage exploration and interest
2. Develop pupil curiosity
3. Cultivate careful observation
4. Provide accurate, firsthand information
5. Clarify concepts and give additional meaning to previous classwork, especially for pupils whose background of experience is very limited
6. Provide opportunities for guidance through direct contact with work opportunities
7. Form new ties between the pupil and his/her community
8. Arouse the interest of parents and other citizens in what schools are doing.

The follow-up activities that result from this field experience include creative projects, class discussions, and the use of other evaluation instruments to measure the understandings gained and the attitudes acquired. The teacher will want to review for him/herself the mechanical and administrative aspects of the trip so that he/she can minimize the difficulties and increase the educational features of future community visits by his/her classes.

RADIO. Radio supplies a certain amount of resource materials that can be timely and vital, and that may have dramatic appeal for the listener. The school broadcast usually is a carefully planned audio-learning experience that utilizes resources beyond those readily available in the classroom. Broadcasts typically are prepared under the supervision of excellent teachers who consult school personnel and subject experts about information that may lend itself to this means of communication. Many topics of personal and community health are in this category.

Wittish and Schuller [3] have identified three rather consistent characteristics of educational radio broadcasts:

1. Educational radio broadcasts provide an immediate awareness
   of and an opportunity for listening participation in current
   history.

2. Educational radio programs make it possible for experts to
   visit classrooms . . . but these become actually team teaching
   demonstrations, with the local teacher as part of the team.

In spite of the desirable features of radio in the classroom, it has
some definite limitations. Among them are:

1. *One-way communication*—During the broadcast, there is no
   opportunity for pupils to ask the radio teacher questions:

2. *Timing*—Adjustment of broadcast time to the specific schedules
   of schools and classes, and adjustment of classwork to the
   actual broadcast time is difficult.

3. *No prehearing or reusability*—The teacher is unable to prehear
   the broadcast. At best he can study the advance announcements
   and the teacher's guide for a particular broadcast.

4. *Lack of nationwide availability*—Not all schools have radios
   or are located with the range of stations that broadcast educational programs.

5. *Poor reception areas*—Some schools are located in areas where
   radio reception is usually of poor quality.

Recordings taken directly off the air or purchased from commercial
sources can be used to overcome most of these limitations. With a disc
or tape recording of a radio broadcast, the teacher does not run the
risk of questionable content, or the inconvenience of set program
schedules. She/he is able to control these factors and can use the
teaching material when it is most desirable and appropriate.

As a first step in the classroom use of radio, the teacher explores
the radio resources that exist in her/his community, and she/he selects
those programs for classroom or home listening that have a direct bear-
ing on current classwork, and that have potential for contributing to
educational outcomes. The subjects of school radio broadcasts are
usually announced well in advance and preliminary study guides are
often provided for teachers so that pupils can be oriented to the experience of listening. Passive listening to radio broadcasts in the classroom
without preplanning, selectivity of the content, and subsequent follow-
up can be a waste of valuable instructional time.

---

[3] Wittish, Walter A., and Schuller, Charles F., *Audiovisual Materials; Their
Nature and Use* (4th Ed.). New York: Harper & Row, 1967. pg. 375.

The significance of radio for teaching discriminative listening has not been fully appreciated. Pupils can be motivated to seek out and critically appraise the various elements that shape up a good radio program, or carefully analyze the accuracy of programs and advertising that contain health information. In the preplanning state, the teacher points up times for listening, and the follow-up activities, which come as a result of the listening experiences, reflect the effectiveness of the broadcast. In addition to classroom listening, pupils can be encouraged to listen at home for radio announcements about current health problems, and to give brief resumes to the class of what they have heard about new advances in medical science, safety precautions, or the work of local health agencies.

The teacher also seek outs opportunities for pupils to participate in actual broadcasts from local stations. When time is granted, the pupils can engage in meaningful activities as they do research, prepare the script, and produce a broadcast based on a health or safety theme. Often pupils' pleas to an adult audience, urging them to take action on some community health problem, bring favorable and immediate response.

RECORDINGS. Tape recording invites exploration as a useful approach to many areas of health and safety education. In some schools, pupils check out tape recorders for class assignments, and return the next day to share the results of a planned interview with, for example, a group of health officials. The tape recorder also may be taken on a field trip to the local health department and a recording made wherever possible of the explanations given during the guided tour. A pupil may choose to record all radio and television commercials with health implications, or programs of health quackery, that can be played back to the class in connection with a unit on consumer health education.

A narrative can be recorded on tape to enhance the showing of a set of school-made slides or a filmstrip on some health or safety topic. A continuous loop of tape can be used by placing, on a strategically located recorder and play-back machine, a message about some health or safety campaign that grows out of a classroom activity.

Many states have duplication centers, each with an extensive collection of permanent recordings on master tapes. A school that orders any of the available recordings sends an appropriate number of blank tapes to the nearest center together with a list of the recordings that are desired. It is an easy process to transfer any recording from one of the master tapes to a school tape. Where outstanding classroom radio programs have been prepared throughout the country, school systems are utilizing tape recordings to exchange programs and to improve the quality of their school-on-the-air broadcasts.

The cassette recorder and tapes certainly have enhanced the possibilities for taping and replaying many worthwhile audio messages.

TELEVISION. A program may be televised: (a) as a live telecast; (b) via video tape, which instantly records both sight and sound on magnetic tape and is ready for immediate use; and (c) on kinescope, which records the live program on motion picture film and which requires processing before it can be used. Video tapes and kinescopes serve much the same purpose for television as recordings do for radio. The main advantage of video tape is that a live program or event can be recorded and played back, with no appreciable loss of quality, a minute, a month, or a year later.

Some telecasting is done on closed circuits. In these instances, the televised information is transmitted by wires, or by microwave, from cameras to private receivers that are located in nearby rooms, buildings, or even at greater distances. In addition to health films for pupils, this type of television is often employed for teacher observation, for teaching manual skills, or to transmit lecture-demonstrations in technical and science courses.

Open-circuit telecasting utilizes the television channels that are controlled and assigned by the Federal Communications Commission. As defined by the Commission, there are two major varieties of television—commercial and educational. Commercial television refers to network programs or those initiated by broadcasting stations that are operated by private organizations primarily for profit. Some of the commercial telecasts have a fairly high educational value, and occasionally they can be used to good advantage in the classroom. Examples of public service programs on commercial television that could be used in a health education class are televised meetings of the World Health Assembly, an illustrated report by a sanitary engineer, a Civil Defense telecast illustrating a new method of resuscitation, and an on-the-spot telecast of antibiotic drug production in a pharmaceutical laboratory.

The Morrill Act of 1862 set aside portions of land in the public domain for educational purposes; on these lands colleges arose. In 1952 the Federal Communications Commission decreed a comparable portion set aside for television. Non-commercial educational television has been the result. Of the programs broadcast on educational channels, some are for out-of-school viewers, while others are for in-school reception and use. Today, school-planned television is a reality, particularly in the centers of heavy population, or close to major universities. The programs are planned and produced by qualified and experienced teachers who work in direct cooperation with school personnel. The programs are developed on topics that have been requested by teachers. Well in advance of each telecast, a copy of the program schedule and its content in the form of teacher and pupil guides is sent to all teachers so that they may prepare their pupils to obtain full benefit from their television experiences.

The designs of educational telecasts vary. Some, especially those for out-of-school viewing, are planned to do the total job of teaching a specific unit of instruction. More frequently, for classroom viewing, the studio teacher provides some basic instruction on a given subject for many pupils in many classrooms. Then, immediately after the telecast, each classroom teacher continues with the same subject, building on the foundation established by the studio teacher and adapting the experience to the needs of individual pupils.

Occasionally, a telecast is used to supplement the regular classwork. For example, by closed circuit, a class that is studying about microorganisms can view a demonstration of an electron microscope in a nearby laboratory. This arrangement enables all of the class members to see the demonstration simultaneously; whereas a field trip to the laboratory not only consumes more time, but pupils have to view the microscope in small groups.

Most often, a live, kinescoped, or video-taped television program is used to enrich classwork. As in selecting any audio-visual material of instruction, the basic questions are: Does the telecast make a contribution to the learning situation beyond that made by instructional materials already in use? Is the general level of the program keyed to the age of the group that will see it? Will the content promote better understanding of the subject? Does the program include useful supplements to the unit of work or the general curriculum area? In answering these questions, the teacher is confronted with the impossibility of previewing a live telecast. In this case, teacher judgment will have to be based on previous experience with the program, the reputation of the sponsor or producer, the caliber of the expert authority or demonstrator who appears on the program, and the care taken in organizing the telecast. These items will help the teacher to decide the probable usefulness of current telecasts and those that may be produced in the future.

Some of the characteristics of television as a teaching device are:

1. *Concreteness of the real and the immediate*—Through the avenues of vision and hearing, television brings the pupil into contact with contemporary events in exciting and clarifying ways. Color sets require even less imagination from viewers.

2. *Uniformity of communication*—Through a television broadcast, teachers, parents, pupils, and citizens may share a common experience at the same time. At least, some essentials may be shared. Beyond that, the influence of the experience depends on the education, experience and interest levels of the individuals.

3. *Succinctness of explanations*—Television has developed a compressed form of communication, whose very succinctness tends to bring clarity. On the other hand, there is always the danger of oversimplification.

4. *Versatility*—Any telecast may use a carefully combined battery of audio-visual materials, such as models, charts, diagrams, exhibits and chalkboards. These add variety and interest, but they can only be viewed by the pupil in the classroom; she/he cannot handle and examine the materials in a televised exhibit.

5. *One-way communication*—Television is primarily a one-way form of communication. The pupils cannot ask questions except where a closed-circuit installation provides microphones for each classroom that permit pupils to communicate with the studio teacher. At present, such talk-back arrangements cannot be made with broadcast television.

MOTION PICTURES. "Hey, it's movie day!" Exclamations such as this herald the probable fact that the sound motion picture is the most frequently used visual aid in health education. The following plus and minus evaluation repeats some of the statements offered for television because, quite obviously, the movie is basically the same as the television program . . . except that the screened picture is grossly larger. Nevertheless, let it be said that educational moving pictures can do the following:

1. Present certain meanings involving motion, sound, information, narration and color (when it is useful) in order to achieve certain understanding

2. Compel and focus attention

3. Increase interest and retention of learning

4. Influence specific attitudes

5. Bring a variety of places and past and current events into the classroom

6. Speed up or slow down time

7. Bring hazardous and difficult demonstrations into the classroom

8. Reduce the size of large objects and, through photomicrography, enlarge things that are too small for the naked eye to see

9. Visualize a concept through animation

10. Clarify relationships among things, ideas and events

11. Provide a satisfying aesthetic experience.

Sound motion films have their limitations, too. Some of them are:

1. The film may contain inaccuracies of fact.

2. The content of a film may become outdated.

3. It is sometimes difficult to obtain a film from a library at the time it would be most helpful.

4. The film may create incorrect concepts of time and size.

5. The film may be too brief or oversimplified.

6. Few films are suitable for all grade levels.

7. The high cost of films prevents many schools from developing their own film libraries.

8. The film may not interest the students.

9. The student may see a school-owned film at various grade levels or in several different classes. Repetitious viewing is boring.

However, films can present skills, action, background information, and facts. In addition, when used by a skilled teacher, they can help build attitudes, stimulate emotions, motivate discussion, and promote critical thinking.

It is best if the teacher can preview a film before showing it to the pupils. Sometimes, because of tight shipping schedules, the teacher may not be able to do so. Study of the excellent teachers' guides that accompany many films will substitute in part for the actual preview, but the teacher is never on safe ground unless the film has been previewed. Sometimes it might be well to omit the use of a film if the teacher has not received it in time for a preview. Some films contain materials that the pupils, and possibly the community, are not prepared to view.

Class preparation is necessary before the film showing to help pupils know what to look for in the film. Otherwise, their purpose in viewing may not be in harmony with the outcomes the teacher hopes to achieve. This is another reason that it is so important for the teacher to preview each film. It is recommended, too, that discussion immediately follow the showing. This may well lead to a variety of other follow-up activities. A greater part of the learning activity follows the film showing.

Step by step, the generally recommended approach would be:

1. Establish the reason for showing the flick.

2. Show the film.

3. Discuss the film as a fulfillment of purposes, and as a stimulus for other learning activities.

4. Reshow the film when necessary to clarify items that may have been missed or only partially comprehended through the initial viewing.

One modification of this procedure consists of stopping the film at a predetermined point and immediately involving the class in discussion of a problem, question, or situation that has been presented by the film.

Following adequate discussion, the rest of the film is shown. Some films are specially designed for this purpose. Another modification is that of individual or small group use of films by pupils. As pupils mature and become experienced in the use of films, under the teacher's guidance, they can conduct previews, screen films to determine if they should be used, develop introductory activities, and plan follow-up procedures.

The loop film, which is approximately 5-to-25 feet of motion picture film, is particularly helpful in teaching difficult skills, and may be utilized with areas of content in which the practice of a given skill is desired while viewing the film. A simple attachment facilitates adaptation to any projector so that a sequence action may be repeated. This technique is particularly useful in teaching first aid and specifically in demonstrating methods of artificial ventilation.

The physical setting and conditions under which a motion picture is viewed determine to a great extent the value of this teaching medium. The regular classroom is a preferred location. It is best if all equipment is set up and ready before the class period begins. Careful attention to the seating arrangements, the ventilation, black-out facilities, the angle of the screen, and proper sound adjustment is required, along with advance assurance that the projector mechanism is in good working order.

One of the criteria for the selection of any teaching aid is that it meets the needs and interests of the particular group with which it is being used. Films prepared for a general audience may not be as effective as those prepared for an audience and a setting of defined characteristics. The magnetic sound projector makes it possible to add a sound track to a locally produced film, to record the commentary, and then to play it back.

Speaking of needs (and we were), the teacher needs to know the types of films available in the health field. Possible helpful categories can be

- Factual or documentary films, with a narrator or some expert, where the purpose is to give facts in a non-dramatic setting
- Story films, where people with names and problems interact with each other, and there is some attempt to generate some identification with and feeling for the subject
- Animated film, serious or humorous, where the picture presentation is other than starkly realistic, perhaps some combination of cartoon and color abstractions. One real advantage of such films is that they do not appear to be out of date as quickly as those with real autos, hair, and clothing styles, etc.
- Trigger or provocative films, designed to create a situation in a few minutes and then leave the viewers with a decision—"What would you do?" or "Well, can you . . . ?"

Many teachers will find of practical value a film evaluation file, which they can keep for future planning and ready reference. The information for each film might be placed on a 3″ by 5″ card, and include a brief summary of the essential points of the film.

There are over 3,000 educational film libraries in the United States. However, the alert teacher acquaints her/himself first with geographically close sources of health films, such as the local and nearby school systems, the state department of education, the local and state health departments, the public library, nearby colleges and universities, and the voluntary health agencies. By studying a variety of film listings, the teacher will find that many films are available at no cost or on loan with only the charge of a return shipping fee. Films obtained from commercial libraries, on the other hand, charge varying rental fees. Since films from local and state sources will usually be in great demand, it is wise to make arrangements well in advance of the showing date.

PROJECTED STILL PICTURES. The filmstrip provides a 35mm film of transparent still pictures or drawings in sequence that may range from 10 to 100 frames on a subject. It is a carefully prepared sequence of teaching material. Filmstrips are available in the silent version and are accompanied by brief explanatory captions or by a script that the teacher can read as each frame is projected on the screen. The sound filmstrip is developed with appropriate commentary and sound effects recorded on a disc or tape. A separate filmstrip projector and a dual-speed record player set at the proper speed will meet the requirements for this type of projection. A special compact projector is available that includes both the projector and record player in one unit. This piece of equipment may also provide for automatic advancing of each frame to correspond with the sound.

The filmstrip has some advantages in that it is compact, relatively inexpensive, can be shown in a semidarkened room, and can be produced locally or within the school to meet a specific need. If the silent version of a filmstrip is used, the teacher is allowed more flexibility since she can easily adapt the material to the pupils in her class. Further, with very little cost, a school or school system can build up its own filmstrip library.

Transparent slides of the 2″ by 2″, or miniature size, and glass or cellophane slides of the standard 3¼″ by 4″ size are other examples of projected still pictures. The slide has characteristics similar to the filmstrip, but provides an added advantage in that the material projected can, but need not, be shown in sequence. Thus, it is possible to select one or two slides to add emphasis or clarity to a particular point in a lesson. Slides can be purchased commercially, or they can be school-made easily and with little cost.

When a teacher has single copies of material or flat objects and wishes to show them to a class, she/he will find opaque projection a useful technique. There is an unlimited variety of opaque material that can be used with this medium of projection. Refinements in the opaque projector have eliminated to a great extent some of its disadvantages in regard to intensity of the light, the cooling system of the apparatus, and the bulk of the projector. Experimentation with the opaque projector will reveal some ingenious uses for this type of teaching aid.

One of the most versatile and useful pieces of hardware for the health education class is the overhead projector. Without darkening the room, the teacher can remain face to face with the class and project prepared transparencies—factual, situational, provocative, or abstract—printed instructions . . . anything that could be written on the chalkboard, but that can be prepared ahead of time. Students can have a learning experience by preparing their own transparencies. A special pen or grease pencil may be used to write or mark on transparencies . . . and all are easily erasable.

Before selecting any of the techniques of still projection described here, the teacher will need to determine whether or not motion is essential to the learning situation. The degree of flexibility that characterizes most still projections can be a distinct advantage in adapting material to the requirements of the group with which it is to be used.

GRAPHIC MATERIALS. There is an abundance of graphic materials from which the teacher can select posters, charts, graphs, maps, diagrams, pictures, comic strips, and cartoons to make her/his teaching more effective. Perhaps the greatest problems confronting the teacher in the use of these materials are filing and cataloguing them so that they will be readily accessible, and evaluating them to ascertain their scientific accuracy and educational soundness.

These media of communication are relatively simple and have optimal usefulness when the focus is on one fact, concept or theme. Because of the degree of abstraction involved, their meaning to the pupils will often be in proportion to the background of experience and information to which they can relate what they see in these pictorial presentations.

Besides providing information, such graphic materials as cartoons and posters can be powerful forces in attitude formation. The choice of a specific type of graphic material depends on the goal that the instructor expects to achieve. The intent may be to motivate pupils to action, to arouse interest or curiosity, to stimulate thinking, to provide factual or comparative data, to influence pupil opinion, or to add humaneness to a problem situation. It is not enough merely to display these materials and leave to chance whatever learning might take place. It is the teacher's responsibility to make certain that the material can be related to something concrete in the learner's experience. If this condition exists, the impact on the observer can be instantaneous and lasting.

There are certain limitations to graphic materials just as there are to all teaching materials. Again, the teacher's competence in selecting and using graphic materials is the guard against misrepresentations, stereotypes, bias, oversimplification, and vague symbolism that may confuse rather than clarify. The potential value of these materials is unlimited if the pupils can be involved in their production and use. They afford an opportunity for pupils with varying degrees of skill and imagination to express their creative talents. The media on which graphic materials can be displayed are the tackboard, the chalkboard, the feltboard and the magnetic board.

Modern and well-planned classrooms reflect consideration for adequate tackboard and chalkboard space. These teaching devices, and their refinements, the feltboard and the magnetic board, offer the teacher countless positive opportunities to mount pictures and symbols to assail the learner's senses.

Today's teacher strives for well-organized and functional displays of graphic material. The principles outlined previously for the use of projected audio-visual materials also apply in the display of graphic materials.

TEXTBOOKS. Textbooks in health education have changed markedly over the years. From an early content of facts and details about the human body, adroitly summarized, but with little functional explanation, the content now typically includes much more usable and realistic information. In contrast to the formerly limited scope of physiology and hygiene, many of the best books now range far into the behavioral, social, physical and ecological sciences to aid the reader in finding solutions to her/his own health problems.

Educators generally agree that with the remarkably rapid growth of knowledge, a body of scientific health information is essential as the core of any health textbook. At the same time, they also agree that the mere statement of authoritative health facts on the printed page is more assurance that the information will be translated into desirable attitudes and health behavior. Textbooks need to be more than encyclopedias. For effective learning, the health information is accompanied by problem-solving experiences in which the knowledge is brought to bear on real life situations.

The teacher plans and prepares to teach with a textbook just as she/he does with any other instructional tool. Authors and publishers give attention to the format and other technical features of the textbook to make it attractive and to capture pupil interest. When used, photographs and other illustrations are carefully selected according to the maturity level and the life context of boys and girls for whom the book is written.

Teachers' manuals or guides provide a wealth of helpful suggestions that the teacher can modify and adapt to her/his classes and pupils. Neither of these are substitutes for good teaching. Pupil workbooks need to be used with caution, lest they become a form of busy work or rote copying from the textbooks. Some current high school workbooks contain health education activities that demand reflective thought by pupils. Wise selection of workbooks is based on their potential motivational power.

In spite of the development and improvement of other instructional materials, the increase in the scope and amount of what is to be learned makes the textbook even more significantly a basic tool in health education. The acknowledged role of books in our society is reflected, too, in the vast selection of paperback volumes that are available to virtually every field of knowledge, including health science. The economical feature of these paperback books makes it possible to enrich the health course immeasurably, and encourages the pupil to do extensive reading on his/her own and to build a library on related topics.

Those responsible for the selection of textbooks and other printed materials are urged to study them carefully for scientific accuracy. Because of the rapid advancements in medical research and allied fields, health education materials need periodic reevaluation with an eye toward elimination and replacement of obsolete items, and selection of those supplementary materials that provide completeness and exactness. Representatives from official, professional and voluntary health organizations can be helpful to teachers in the task of judging health education materials for their adherence to currently accepted facts.

SOURCES OF ASSISTANCE, INFORMATION AND MATERIALS. The health teacher is expected to help her/his students understand how the latest discoveries in the medical and health sciences relate to their behaviors. This requires much more than merely imparting knowledge. The teacher's task is to create an opportunity for a full range of learning, attitudes, and feelings, as well as information. Health teaching necessarily draws on many sciences for the best information on how to live, and on the broad field of education for skills to make this information meaningful. Thus, the teacher has to look to others for specialized knowledge and enrichment materials that will strengthen her/his teaching. She/he looks first within the school, next within the community, and then outside the community.

RESOURCES WITHIN THE SCHOOL. Many schools have developed teachers' guides that include classified listings of the audio-visual materials, resource persons and agencies, textbooks, pamphlets, and other health education resources that are readily available. The teacher needs to know what materials and equipment, such as projectors, charts and models, are in her/his building and what may be secured through the central office.

Many school systems provide health education materials through the school or public library. Periodicals, pamphlets, films, slides and recordings, as well as books, are provided. Many libraries carry current catalogues of audio-visual suppliers and listings of films, posters and pamphlets that are available locally. The teacher can locate further leads in the card catalogues; indexes such as the *Education Index, Readers' Guide to Periodical Literature, Educational Film Guide, Catalogue of Free Teaching Aids, Selected United States Government Publications,* and other sources for locating up-to-date information and audio-visual materials. The school librarian is a helpful resource person for teachers who are seeking aids to better teaching.

SCHOOL STAFF RESOURCES. Some school systems have a director of curriculum or a coordinator of audio-visual materials who heads a centralized service apart from the library. Some county school offices also include an audio-visual department. One function of the director or coordinator of these departments is to assist teachers in securing curriculum materials for classroom use.

A specialist in health education may be employed. She/he may teach some health classes and devote part of her/his time to the promotion of a complete school health program. Her/his title may be health consultant, coordinator, supervisor, or director of health education. Each elementary school and high school may have a teacher appointed to serve as coordinator of health education. The helpfulness of these people in providing source materials and information depends on their qualifications, interest, time and assigned responsibilities.

There may be a variety of health specialists working on the school health team who can be called on from time to time to help teachers with special problems. The school medical adviser, the nurse who serves the school, the dentist, dental hygienist, nutritionist, and speech and hearing therapist expect to serve as resource persons. The teacher may ask these people to help her/him find materials and keep her/him informed about the newer knowledge of their health specialties. There may be times when it is desirable to have these specialists serve as resource visitors to the classroom.

RESOURCES WITHIN THE COMMUNITY. Within the community, the teacher will find official and non-official health agencies such as city or county health departments, voluntary health associations, and professional organizations, such as the local medical and dental societies.

The local health department, if a fully qualified unit organized at the county or city level, is a most helpful source of information and materials. The modern health department recognizes education as a means for preventing and ameliorating today's community health problems, and it is usually staffed to carry on a public health education program. Many health departments employ health educators who assist in the schools when they are invited to do so. In some instances, a health educator is employed jointly by the departments of education and health with the school health education program as her/his major responsibility.

Ideally, the full-time local health department has at least a medical health officer, a sanitary officer, a laboratory technician, a clerk, and a public health nurse on its professional staff. Larger units may have health educators, public health dentists, dental hygienists, nutritionists, and other specialists. The clerk can usually direct the teacher to proper personnel for the help she/he needs. The health department sometimes provides the school with health services. Where this is done, public health nurses make periodic visits to the school. At this time they are usually willing to discuss with the teacher health instruction materials as well as the health problems of certain children. The teacher cannot afford to overlook other branches of local government, such as the police and fire departments and environmental protection agencies, as sources for materials and consultants in certain aspects of health and safety education.

Voluntary health agencies provide education and service as part of their programs. The better known agencies are well-organized at either the city or county level. Voluntary health agencies have been active in the development of public health programs in this country since the early part of the present century. Each is concerned with special health problems. They raise money for research and experimental programs, and support the activities of official health agencies. A major objective of these organizations is the education of the community about specific health needs. The teacher usually will find local chapters of the voluntary health agencies concerned with cancer, lung problems, heart diseases, prevention of blindness, hearing conservation, and other specific health problems. Often they can furnish her/him with films, filmstrips, teaching guides, and up-to-date printed information concerned with their special areas. These materials usually have been developed by the state or national offices of the agencies, but can be secured more quickly, free, or at lower cost through the local units.

Voluntary agencies have served the schools well by furnishing teaching aids, helping in the preparation of teachers' guides, assisting with short-term projects, promoting the in-service education of teachers, providing speakers and consultants for pupils and teachers, and participating on school health committees. Considerable attention has been given to the ways through which voluntary agencies may work cooperatively in the school health program.

Local medical, dental and other professional societies are interested in school health education and services, and in recent years many of them have formed school health committees to help schools improve their programs. Most of the materials available through the local professional organizations have been developed at the state and national levels. Resource people from these organizations can assist in special areas of health instruction such as home nursing, quackery, drug and sex education. Representatives from these groups can also be helpful in the scientific evaluation of health education materials, and as members of the school health council.

In recent years, schools, colleges and communities have formed health councils to mobilize their health resources in ways that will best serve the school and community. Such councils provide opportunities for lay and professional people to exchange ideas and information. Through studies and surveys, the health council can determine the most important health needs of a school or community. The chairman of a health council can advise the teacher where to get help on certain problems.

RESOURCES OUTSIDE THE COMMUNITY. When the health teacher seeks health education assistance, information and materials outside the school system and local community, she/he finds a large number of sources that lead to a core of authentic and reliable enrichment materials.

Most state departments of education have consultants in school health. These people are employed to help school systems improve their health education programs. Also, most states have minimum standards and legal requirements for health and safety instruction in schools. Usually the state department of education provides guides for elementary and secondary health teaching, as well as pamphlets, films, and other teaching materials on health topics. The growing trend through comprehensive health education legislation often provides more guides and state frameworks for teacher use.

State health departments often have specialists in maternal and child health, disease control, dental health, sanitation, nutrition, mental health and health education. Films, bulletins, pamphlets and other materials are available for school use. The state health departments may prefer that school personnel channel requests for materials or consultant services through the school superintendent and the local health department or district office. Both state and local health departments can be helpful in securing teaching materials from national sources.

Services for schools from state departments of health and education have been improved in recent years by joint planning between the two departments. Such planning permits the employment of specialists to serve both departments, provides coordinated services, eliminates duplication of materials, and avoids confusion by following common policies for school health programs. Some states have planning committees or councils that not only include representatives from the state departments of health and education, but also from voluntary health agencies, professional societies, and teacher preparation institutions.

The U.S. Department of Health, Education and Welfare at the national level has been in a state of periodic reorganization since the late 1960's. It has several important services for schools. Since it has never been clear whether health education should be considered under health or under education (and these two are separated in the Department), neither has taken this on as a major responsibility. Whatever is written about H.E.W. at this time probably would not be accurate or complete when you read this. So, check and see what present conditions are.

The National Education Association is a professional organization of educators. It works with other groups to improve education through better schools and advancement of the professional, economic, social and civic status of teachers. Through its affiliated state associations, the N.E.A. represents the concerns of millions of teachers. It publishes *Today's Education* and hundreds of other journals, bulletins, books and pamphlets devoted to the interests of teachers and the promotion of better education at all levels. One of N.E.A.'s affiliates, the American Alliance for Health, Physical Education and Recreation, publishes *Health Education,* a periodical focused entirely on school health education, and numerous other bulletins, pamphlets and books in school health education and related fields.

The Joint Committee on Health Problems in Education of the National Education Association and the American Medical Association is a committee of representatives from both the medical and education professions that has functioned since 1911. In addition to its publication, *Health Education,* the Committee has published two other books, *School Health Services* and *Healthful School Environment.* The sex education series (four booklets) and "Health Appraisal of School Children" are among the many publications of this Committee. These publications can be secured from the American Medical Association or the National Education Association.

The American Medical Association and its state, territorial, county and city medical societies have a deep interest in school, college and public health education. The Association publishes the *Journal of the American Medical Association, Prism, AMA News,* speciality journals for its members, *Today's Health,* which interprets medical opinion on health problems to lay people, *Health Education Service for Schools and Colleges,* a monthly four pager of abstracted articles on youth in health and non-health, and *More Life for Your Years,* a monthly newsletter. *Today's Health* and *Health Education Service* are valuable resources for teachers at all levels and for health classes at the secondary and college levels. The AMA has a Department of Health Education staffed by health educators, physicians and other personnel to promote school and public health. Through this and other departments, and in conjunction with other organizations, the Association has developed valuable resource materials.

Among the best avenues to reliable, current information and new materials are the American Alliance for Health, Physical Education and Recreation; The American School Health Association; and the School Health Section of the American Public Health Association. These professional organizations are concerned primarily with school health. They publish journals that, besides having articles on various aspects of health education, carry book reviews, news from the field, annotated bibliographies and notices of new teaching materials. These groups have annual meetings at which members gather to discuss new knowledge in health science and health education. They have affiliated state and, in some instances, district or regional organizations that also meet periodically.

School health problems are of interest to many of the numerous sections of the American Public Health Association, but since its organization in 1942, the School Health Section has attempted to bring together those with particular interests in school health education. The Section functions throughout the year by means of committees that are appointed to study and report on certain health problems. Committee reports, many of which have direct implications for health teaching, are published in the *American Journal of Public Health* and/or *The Nation's Health,* the Association's monthly newspaper.

The American School Health Association has a membership that includes physicians, dentists, dental hygienists, school nurses, optometrists, nutritionists, podiatrists, health educators, and school administrators. The Association has many study committees that prepare recommendations and reports on all phases of school health. The Committee reports and a variety of health education articles are published in the *Journal of School Health.*

Since 1931, the American Academy of Pediatrics has had a Committee on School Health that gives special attention to school health services. Reports of the Committee are printed in *Pediatrics,* a monthly publication of the Academy. This has encouraged the active participation of pediatricians in school health services, and has given schools the benefit of their thinking on health education problems. Reprints of the Committee's reports are available on request. The Academy has a variety of publications on school health.

The American Dental Association has a strong interest in health education of the public. Its Bureau of Dental Health Education has developed excellent resource materials for schools and offers consultation services. A listing of its literature, special publications, and audiovisual materials is available upon request.

The voluntary health agencies at the state and national levels are interested in health education. At state and national levels, the programs of these associations are similar in organization and methods of education, while local level programs are varied to meet community needs. These associations develop and distribute excellent pamphlets, teaching guides, plays, charts, and posters for school use. As previously indicated, teachers can save time and sometimes money by securing these materials through the local units.

Commercial organizations have developed some most worthwhile and attractive health education materials. Many life insurance companies and industry-sponsored associations produce extensive amounts of enrichment materials that are accurate and free of objectionable advertising. Many private companies supply materials of excellent quality at no cost and with no more advertising than an identifying label. On the other hand, some manufacturers and distributing companies mislead the public in order to sell their products. Their educational materials are not suitable for classroom use.

The following criteria are helpful in evaluating the health instructional materials prepared by commercial organizations:

1. The material should bear a clear, but modest, label identifying its source.
2. It should be free from advertising.
3. It should be scientifically accurate.
4. It should be consistent with modern educational methodology.
5. It should not promote products, services, or concepts that are contrary to accepted good health principles and practices.

Consultants from the local health department, voluntary health agencies and the county medical society can be helpful to individual teachers and to teacher committees in applying these criteria.

In the international realm, the International Union for Health Education still survives and publishes the *International Journal of Health Education* in three languages and holds regular world conferences.

RESOURCE FILE OF TEACHING MATERIALS. If the health teacher is going to make full use of the tremendous amount of available reference and teaching materials, it becomes necessary for her/him to develop a simple, flexible resource file. As the teacher reads articles, pamphlets and books that are valuable to her/him, she/he makes notations of certain information on filing cards. The use of separate cards permits alphabetical arrangement by topics. Each card carries a brief resume of the contents, merit, and use of a given item. For books and pamphlets the essentials include: author's name, complete title, place of publication, name of publisher, date of publication, and cost. For periodicals they include: author's name, title of article, name of journal, number of volume, date of publication, and numbers of the pages on which the article appears.

A card file for films and other audio-visual materials can be developed. Here, each card contains how, where and the time needed to secure the material, as well as its cost. Other useful information to note depends on the nature of the material. Through annotation of lesson plans, the teacher can note how any one item is used and how it might be used again. It is important to replace notations on out-of-date materials, especially pamphlets and films, with current ones on more recent items.

The health teacher cannot keep all of the materials that come to her/his attention. However, she/he can develop the ability to scan and recognize what is useful, according to the guidelines presented in this and other chapters. A resource file is basic for good planning and efficient use of teaching materials.

SUMMARY BY A ROUND TABLE OF EDUCATORS: "I use films and filmstrips regularly in my teaching of tenth graders, and always as a planned part of a unit. By the end of a term, my students recognize the different styles and purposes of films and are not only more informed on health issues but are more aware of how these audio-visuals help us learn."

"Third and fourth graders need to see things to really learn. In my health teaching, I do some demonstrations, have exhibits and bulletin board displays all through the year, and take my class to the health museum once each term."

"The overhead projector and visual transparencies constitute my favorite audio-visual method. Rather than use a wide variety, I am trying to develop many ways of using this aid in helping my ninth graders learn."

"Through the dental society we got in touch with a dental hygienist who is particularly interested in helping young children become more aware of how they can take care of their teeth. She has talked to our kindergarten and first-grade classes, she has a wonderful approach to children, and we see her as a tremendous learning resource."

"My classes of twelfth graders check the television guide at the beginning of each week and decide which programs, documentary or dramatic or whatever, potentially apply to health. Then they try to make sure some students, at least, watch each program selected. Some Fridays we take time to discuss and analyze some of the programs. We don't build the course around them, but they're a pretty regular supplementary resource . . . and this practice tends to make my students more aware of the health implications in television programs."

"One of my eighth-grade health teachers uses a film every Friday . . . a full period film with little or no discussion. The films are usually good, but they may not relate to what was studied during the week. The teacher is tenured, and this practice, in effect, gives him Fridays off."

"We had a guest speaker recommended by one of our community agencies, and he was *awful!* He was not only a waste of time, but was a detriment to what I was trying to get across."

"As the coordinator for teaching-learning resource materials in this district, I would say some teachers misuse some of the resource materials, but the majority of teachers try to improve the learning in their classes. My problem is how to decide how to use my time and that of my staff to keep materials current, moving and evaluated and how to spend the funds we have to accomplish the most learning."

Chapter XIV

So What Have We Accomplished? (Sometimes Tabbed *Evaluation*)

SOME KNOWLEDGE IS MORE IMPORTANT THAN SOME OTHER. I was talking to a man the other day who just had completed a 100-hour course in emergency medical treatment as a special qualification for being a volunteer fireman. Out of a class of 13, he told me that he was the only person to pass the final exam and therefore the course. Though everyone passed the academic portion of the exam, all but Tom goofed on the practical-situational emergency. He was the only one who thought to check for a possible broken neck, and therefore, in the instructor's judgment, his classmates, though ministering well otherwise, potentially killed their accident victims.

In an examination this past spring, I asked students to compare and contrast self-actualization (as a Western cultural mental health concept) and self-realization (as an equally important Eastern cultural mental health concept) as they would be manifested in two personalities, Abner and Punya. About half of the students wrote excellent to adequate comparisons . . . according to my judgment.

Consider these as two illustrations of one important principle of evaluation in health education: there is a range in the critical nature of health learnings . . . from life or death matters to very esoteric, general knowledge learnings, but such distinctions may not be clear to the learners. That is, the instructor's action in the first example is not a common one. Rather, the typical health exam is a mixture of critical and picayune matters, but all with the same number of points . . . and the same passing grade can result from missing many critical points or missing items of much lesser importance.

Two situations point up another important principle:

I wanted students to be able to distinguish between narcotics and other dangerous drugs in two different ways (legal and pharmacological) and to present one argument for and one argument against the legalization of marijuana. Ninety-two percent of my students were able to do this satisfactorily after our study of drugs.

The study of drug use and abuse in my seventh-hour class developed into consideration of the bigger issue of personal responsibility and social control of irresponsible persons. The students didn't learn much new about drugs, but ninety-two percent were able to identify the philosophical assumptions behind various approaches to controlling abuse.

The principle: there are two general purposes for evaluation

    a. to assess to what extent objectives were achieved

    b. to assess what else happened and what other things were learned.

If a teacher has objectives, she/he wants to know how well they are achieved. In addition, a dynamic class atmosphere may bring about other learnings—some important, some trivial, and some embarrassingly counter to what "should have been." A teacher wants to know these other consequences of the learning game.

PROCESS AS WELL AS CONTENT. Sometimes assessment of growth and progress is thought of mainly in terms of content . . . ideas, concepts, facts learned. Recall one major thrust of this volume: health education is both content and process. Translated to the present concern, this calls for evaluating not only what students have learned, but also how well they have learned to learn.

Are students able to prepare for and execute a debate? . . . participate actively in a symposium? . . . evaluate a film? . . . interpret a visual transparency (or other picture)? . . . dramatize a decision-making situation or interpret the dramatization? . . . distinguish between a legitimate and a less legitimate authority? . . . Though some assessment of these ways of functioning may be made, they tend to be observational and superficial and rarely a significant contributor to any given grade. This tends to communicate to learners that "what" is considerably more important than "how." And is it really?

CHANGE BEHAVIOR? One of the unexamined beliefs of the health education field is that the central aim is to change behavior. As noted in earlier pages, this assumes that all pre-health education behavior is undesirable and in need of change. It should be obvious that this is not true, and the aim must be the more ambiguous one of changing some behavior and reinforcing other practices. Behavior is influenced by what an individual knows (from all sources) and what his motives, attitudes, and predispositions are. Education purposes to change or reinforce selectively in these realms. However, this raises another question, Should it be this or should it be that kind of question about evaluation? Should evaluation try to determine what a person knows, feels, and does that is different from her/his pre-instruction state of being OR should it merely assess what a person knows, feels, and can do without concern for where or how it was learned? If "Yes" is the answer to the first alternative, there must be rather extensive pre-testing, reliably related to the final evaluation and to the modes of instruction.

How Do Teachers Feel About Pre-Testing?

- I always give a pre-test on each unit. It tells me what a class knows and doesn't know, and gives me a clear direction for the instruction in the unit.
- I periodically give a pre-test to check my judgments, but generally I come pretty close to predicting what they know and what they don't . . . without a formal test.
- I sometimes give a pre-test, but instruction time is so limited that I'm inclined to skip it and get on with the teaching-learning.
- A good pre-test for a whole concept has to be so long it gets boring. Instead of stimulating behavior, it often does the opposite. And just a short pre-test doesn't seem worth giving.
- I used to give pre-tests, but I got very frustrated in deciding what to do with the results. If 70 percent of a class knows something that is important or has a constructive attitude, should I strive to raise this to 90 or 100 percent . . . or should I concentrate on something less important that few students know . . . or on some lesser attitude?
- I associate pre-testing with research, and I feel, rightly or wrongly, that teaching and research are different bags. For this reason, it just doesn't seem right for me to pre-test.

And so it goes. Most teachers understand the reasons for pre-testing, but I suspect (in lieu of any clear research study to give a verifiable answer) that not many consistently give the pre-measure to determine exactly where students are. Whatever the reasons for not giving the pre-instruction evaluation, the fact that it is not given means there might not be an accurate measuring of the effects of the classroom learning.

Learning is a fairly complex phenomenon involving interactions among (1) new ideas to be learned, (2) older ideas to be reinforced, (3) retention and (4) forgetting. Therefore, it is never terribly clear whether something that is known before health instruction is forgotten in the process of learning something else, or whether reinforcing the learning, particularly through some application, insures its retention for a longer period of time than would have been so without the repeat.

AHA! PREVENTION. Much health education, as it is translated into young Sam's and Sally's behavior (or non-behavior), is supposed to be a factor in prevention of some potential problems or difficulty. Yet, prevention is often not easily evaluated. If something is prevented, it does not happen . . . right? But would it have happened if the preventive measure—e.g., education—had not occurred? The most general evaluation of drug education programs in the early 1970's is that they were ineffective. Sam and Sally were in a health course with a drug education segment, and a year later neither is a drug user. Was the course effective? In a gross way it was, because drug use was prevented . . . true? Ah, but would Sam and Sally have been non-users anyway? There is no way to know for sure. Probabilities are the best means of prognosis available. Characteristics of users and non-users can be compared and contrasted, and these probability models correlated with traits manifested by Sam and Sally. Let's pretend that these various judgments can be finally quantified and that the comparison suggested that Sam had a 20 percent chance of being a drug user and Sally a 75 percent chance. That would seem to indicate that the education was more effective for Sally since prevention of use was more unlikely in her case. What other factors were operating? In what ways did some things learned reinforce other forces, rather than prevent de novo?

A DIFFICULT EVALUATION. Such an attempt at evaluation . . . to determine exactly to what extent some aspects of the classroom education experience did prevent Sam and Sally from becoming drug users . . . obviously is difficult, if not impossible. If it were finally and carefully done for Sally and Sam, would it be of any value for Jack and Shirley and the other four million or so youngsters in their age group?

This seems to be a put-down of evaluations, and it really is not intended to be. It is intended as a counter to rather simplistic cries to determine if health education is effective or not. The answer to such a question is nearly as much a function of assumptions and values as it is of measurable results. And it probably always will be.

CLASSROOM AND NON-CLASSROOM BEHAVIOR. The examples used thus far perhaps point up an important characteristic of that to be evaluated in health education. As in several other analyses of the field, I would propose these as polar extremes of a continuum rather than clearly dichotomous categories:

- Evaluation of classroom behavior (such as writing a paper, answering test questions, performing in a sociodrama, evaluating a film. . . .)
- Evaluation of outside-of-school personal behavior (such as smoking grass, fasting, driving an automobile safely, kissing infected friends, overcoming feelings of social inadequacy. . . .)

BEHAVIOR NOT GRADED. Much of the behavior to which the content of a health course translates occurs outside of the classroom, out of the schoolhouse, or after the course has been completed. Little direct evaluation of such is practical. Oh, some behavior, of course, is observable in the classroom or around school—things like food selection, carrying a pack of cigarettes, verbal relations with other students, going to sleep in class, control of temper, care of a running nose . . .—but evaluation is rarely more than observational. That is, there are jokes and cartoons on the theme that the unmarried girl who gets pregnant flunks her sex education class. This implies grading on actual behavior. Rarely is this truly considered appropriate as even an influence on the grade. Sally and Sam are graded on performance in typing, in music, in art, in shop, in swimming . . . but in health they are graded on what they know and say they would do about healthy performance. Why? Because health-related behavior is often very personal, and in our culture social institutions are not to mess up an individual's personal behavior—unless she/he desires such or unless the individual has acted irresponsibly toward others. Considering the above non-health examples, it is generally easier to grade on typing performance than on artistic performance, since the latter has many more personal dimensions. It is easier to grade on actual swimming speed and endurance than on form and style, again because of personal preference dimensions.

Another reason is that much healthy behavior simply increases potentials for, rather than guarantees, better living performances. A smoker still may win the 100-yard dash; a person eating beautifully balanced meals still may get the flu; and a lad very discriminating about sexual partners still may contact syphilis. So, we know what's healthy, but our evaluative criteria are not as firm as we would like them to be.

CLASSROOM EVALUATION. Meanwhile, back in the classroom . . . how are learners evaluated? Well, they perform tangible tasks, like taking tests, writing papers and doing projects, and the teacher grades these, using criteria that may range from the very definite and clear to the very personal and subjective. They self-report certain activities (watching a television documentary, interviewing a dental hygienist, observing traffic patterns at a particularly dangerous corner . . .) that indicate interest, motivation and potential learnings. They are observed by the teacher in such settings as a small discussion group, listening to another student's report, interacting with other students before and after class, playing a sociodrama role. . . .

INDIVIDUALISTIC AND COMPETITIVE. Students can also evaluate one another, of course. Many obviously do . . . and often . . . in order to form their own judgments. Some teachers encourage peer evaluation, but relatively few seem to trust these enough to include them in the official evaluation for the course. Some feel students tend to be too easy on one another . . . or on friends. Others perceive that they may be too hard on classmates. Of course, the main orientation of American education is individualistic and competitive, and students competing against one another are not exactly encouraged to make fair judgments on fellow learners. Also, some see getting high grades as not necessarily related to learning, so any way to get a higher grade is worth trying.

In contrast to this spirit, some of the first reports on education coming out of the People's Republic of China in the early 1970's [1,2] portrayed an overwhelming emphasis on cooperation. In one report on higher education, the point was made that no grades were given. The answer to the question, How, then, would you know who was the ablest physicist in a class? is easily answered by asking the members of the class . . . they know best. Building on this cultural contrast, it occurred to me that while cheating is generally defined in American education as not doing your own, individual work, the Chinese definition might well be giving an answer that you have kept to yourself and not shared with the other members of the class.

WHAT THEY KNOW . . . OR DON'T KNOW. All evaluation activities have educational value, but some are designed to be real learning experiences in themselves. Others tend toward assessing only what has been learned. Another interesting range in emphasis is the extent to which any constructed test tries to find out what takers of it know in contrast to what they do not know. Test construction theory holds that a desirable test item is one that differentiates between the able and the less able; consequently, an item that everyone gets right is not a desirable test item. But one of Mr. Fry's main objectives is to have all students know that, at this time, there are two fundamental ways of preventing the contraction of venereal disease—(a) not having sexual intercourse or other intimate relations with an infected person and (b) the proper male use of a reputably manufactured condom. Mr. Fry wants to know whether everyone does finally know this. He is pleased if every student gets it correct. He sees answering the question as a positive reinforcement of learning that he wants to last as long as possible. This would be an example of an evaluation that is clearly related to the learning objectives and measures the extent to which students learn something they are supposed to know.

Mr. Graybo, a colleague of Mr. Fry's, takes an opposite tack. His comparable question is, "Name the three venereal diseases other than syphilis and gonorrhea (and they must be spelled correctly)." These were not mentioned in class, but were in the textbook. The better students know he will ask something like this, so they have memorized a hoard of little details. The rest of the class just doesn't bother . . . each does the best she/he can to get a few things correct. Relatively few get full credit, and about 30 percent get no credit at all on this question. It is a good differentiator. But how worthy is the knowledge?

----

[1] Mirsky, Jonathan, "A Sinologist in China," *Saturday Review of the Society*, 55:48 (No. 27), July 1, 1972.

[2] Swetz, Frank J., "Chinese Education and the Great Cultural Revolution," *Contemporary Education*, 44:159 (No. 3), January 1973.

WHAT DO THEY KNOW? More importantly, the majority of Mr. Graybo's students have shown him that they do not know the other three venereal diseases, but he still does not know what they do know.

True-false questions are the worst examples of this not knowing what they know syndrome. A test item might be:

T or F. The amount of alcohol consumed is the only factor in how drunk an individual may be.

False is the correct answer, but the teacher does not then know what correct answerers think other factors might be. (Joe knows that time spent drinking is the other major factor; Harold thinks the amount of self-discipline and moral character is the other big one.) Another item might be:

T or F. Behavior modification is a basis for therapy in mental illness in which the emphasis is on getting the patient to behave more normally.

Students marking this true would display some acquaintance with the behavior modification theory. What do those who mark it false believe?

MISCONCEPTIONS. This leads to another interesting and important observation about wrong answers—or misconceptions, as they usually are called in the research literature. Some misconceptions are crucial and should be vigorously corrected. If Gordon believes that:

. . . In an emergency medical situation (accidental injury), the first thing to do is call a physician.

Gordon could allow someone to die of bleeding or suffocation while doing what he knows to be best. If Sheila believes that:

. . . the safe period is that six or eight days midway between the menstrual periods

Sheila might find herself nourishing a new, unwanted, embarrassing life within her womb.

Still other misconceptions invoke a cry of So what! My favorite is that some students think you should take left-over food out of the original cans to store it in the refrigerator. If they act on this misconception, is there likely to be any ill-health? Pretty clearly no.

GRADING. By the fourth or fifth grade, evaluation seems quite objective and exact. Students perform various kinds of tasks, and teachers assign numbers or letters or both so that these can be translated into a grade. For example, a ninth-grade teacher might report:

Johnny got a 67 on the first exam and a 53 on the second; he got a C+ on his project and he accumulated 137 points on daily work and class participation; he scored 125 on the final. He earned a C− for the semester.

Obviously, these numbers are meaningless unless we know the total possible points. Then it generally is the individual teacher's judgment as to what some point total represents. As in the above example, Johnny's teacher gives him a C−, which will become part of his official transcript, and forever after it can be verified, by a notarized copy, that Johnny got a C− in health in his freshman high school year. This could become part of the basis for deciding whether he is qualified for a job when he is 34 years old. It really is rather silly, but we are generally a culture that respects quantification, and no better system seems agreeable or workable, so grade assignment continues.

WHICH IS BEST? The obvious question from conscientious professionals should be, Which form of evaluation is best . . . most valid? The obvious question from busy teachers probably is, Which form of evaluation is easiest . . . takes the least time . . . is easiest to translate into grades? Hospitals and clinics have to be run in many respects for the staff in order that busy professionals do not waste time and energy in determining what's going on. Schools and classrooms, too, are organized to waste a minimum of professional teacher time. Obviously there are differences of opinion between some administrators and some members of their staffs on what is the best procedure.

First, there probably is no keen answer to the request for best. The more objective the type of evaluation, the more the learner is required to indicate knowledge in circumscribed set ways. The more the form allows free student expression, the more subjective the evaluation becomes and the more thinking like the teacher is likely to be rewarded. Actually, virtually any question worth its salt has subjective elements to it. True-false, multiple-choice, matching, or fill-in questions have subjectivity built into the question and the choices offered. The correct answer is (c), and all others are wrong; that is because the question writer has subjectively cut down the possibilities to those given. She/he says, in effect, I don't care what else you know about this subject, just see if you agree with me on this point. The essay question, on the other hand, shifts the subjectivity to the actual answer written. How does the teacher who gave students some leeway in how they could answer actually judge and compare the various answers . . . with her own . . . with others answering the same question . . . with remembrances of how students have answered in past years . . .? She probably may not know . . . just knows what is right . . . or good.

DIFFERENT ABILITIES AND RESPONSES. More importantly, however, the best question has no real answer because the principle developed for learning activities applies also to evaluations. Different learners respond well to different approaches, and no approach brings forth equally satisfying results from all learners. In my experience at the undergraduate college level, the easiest way to get a normal curve distribution of grades for a class is to give one type of evaluation all the way through, with no credit for any other evidence of learning. Those who do well on this type of test are reinforced and continue to do well (even improve), while those who do not do well are reinforced in their mediocrity and tend to try less hard. In contrast, I have found that the more different (really different) forms of evaluation I employ, the harder it is to give low grades . . . and, interestingly, it is also not as easy to differentiate the superior students, for I have found some ways in which the excellent orthodox student cannot perform well. If this is true in a college class, where students have come through a formal and informal selection process and they all are humans who can learn by reading and listening and can perform well on tests, it should be even more true in a school classroom. This observation gives me the uneasy feeling that our notions about a range in actual learning is, to some extent, a self-fulfilling prophecy. If good teaching or good evaluation is supposed to produce 35 percent C's, then some students just have to be the C students. And one consistent type of evaluation (a select answer test requiring above average reading ability) seems to be the most efficient way to produce this standard.

MEANS OF EVALUATION. All right, let's review some means that are or can be used to evaluate learners in health. The examples below present some advantages and some disadvantages . . . from the standpoint of the teacher and learner.

TEST QUESTIONS

Where Learners Select Answers

Advantage	Disadvantage
Learner: You have some clues that can help you remember.	*Learner:* You have to read each carefully because one word may be the difference between right and wrong.
Teacher: Easy to correct.	*Teacher:* Good questions of this type take time to construct.

Where Learners Provide Answers

Advantage	Disadvantage
Learner: You can express yourself more freely . . . you can 'work in' the things you know.	*Learner:* It may not be clear just what the teacher wants . . . I can write what I think is a good answer, but the teacher had something else in mind.
Teacher: As a student builds a fairly complex answer, it can become evident how she/he is thinking and what she/he knows about the subject.	*Teacher:* Students who really don't know the answer can wander around trying to say something relevant . . . judgments are often difficult in giving partial credit for some good ideas.

Written Papers Or Reports

Advantage

Learner: If you can select your own topic, you can really get into and learn something that you're interested in.

Disadvantage

Learner: Some people just can't write papers . . . sometimes the topic isn't that interesting . . . sometimes there are not resource materials . . . frustrating. The grade is the teacher's subjective judgment.

Creative Projects

Advantage

Learner: These can really get you to think . . . and allow you to express some ideas in different— even 'far-out'—ways.

Teacher: A good creative project not only can indicate how a student understands and can apply an idea or a concept, but it also can give you, the grader, some new insights.

Disadvantage

Learner: These can take a lot of time . . . and you're never sure you're really on the right track . . . they also can be pretty Mickey Mouse . . . and the grading is very subjective.

Teacher: Some students just cannot express creatively. It is very hard to downgrade a student for expressing an idea in a very ordinary, prosaic way . . . then, some students are more creative than the teacher, and it is embarrassing not to understand what the student meant to convey.

Group Work

Teacher: A group that works well together can present the best combination of the knowledge and talents of members . . . and the experience is a good one for students to evaluate one another. It is a means of learning that an individual may not always be evaluated on her/his own work alone.

Teacher: In evaluating a group project, it is never possible to know the value of each individual's contribution. An individual may be penalized by being in a group that just does not function well together.

Oral Question and Answer

Advantage

Learner: This is the main way we're going to have to use whatever ideas we have after the class is over . . . some people do not write well, but they can 'think on their feet' and answer a question very well . . . such kinds should get credit for this ability.

Disadvantage

Learner: Answering a question under pressure in front of the whole class can be embarrassing . . . so that you really don't answer at your best . . . some people don't speak well and shouldn't be graded on whether they can or not.

Some other means of evaluations with brief annotations . . .

Discuss and Write. Advantageous to those who can express themselves in writing . . . gives the teacher an opportunity to judge what all members of a class have learned.

Observing Students. Gives some valuable personal insights . . . these may be difficult to translate to a tangible number or letter . . . not always possible to note behavior tangibly when it occurs (must remember!) . . . students' behavior may or may not represent their real state of learning. . . .

Videotaping. Allows unlimited playback for fair evaluation of student performance . . . but is just not available on a regular basis to be used as needed in most schools.

Analysis of a Picture. Pictures may be more realistic stimuli than words for many learners . . . more difficult to justify not giving credit for an answer that appears wrong or inappropriate to teacher, but not to student.

The reader's imagination and experience can provide other media with appropriate pros and cons.

CHEATING . . . AGAIN. Somewhere earlier in this chapter, we puttered around for a bit with the matter of cheating and how it is culturally defined. Let's look a bit more closely at this culture and try to see both why cheating occurs and why it does not occur more often. Also, let's explore why the evaluator is responsible for a considerable amount of cheating. As already stated, the predominant ethos of the educational system is individualistic and competitive. Each individual receives grades on his/her individual performance as it is compared with that of others. There are only so many A's, and a certain number of unsatisfactory grades are expected. In a class of 230 where there is a class ranking, there is a person who is No. 1 and, finally, a person who is No. 230. Students are taught that they are not to cheat, which means that they are to submit only their work and judgments. They must remember all kinds of things without outside help (crib sheets, ponies, answers or abbreviations on the inside of the wrist, etc.) To be caught cheating typically results in losing all credit for work legitimately done. Anti-cheating tends to be supported by the naturally successful portion of any class, because the advantage gained by the cheater could be to their disadvantage.

TEACHER AS CHEATER ENCOURAGER. The teacher as evaluator enters the picture by (a) giving a type of exam on which it is easy to cheat (true-false, multiple choice, short answer) and/or (b) asking too many questions to which students do not know the answers. "Cheating seems less wrong in Miss Crow's class . . . what she asks really isn't fair . . . has almost nothing to do with what we've been studying." So, to the extent that teachers ask students to recall burdensome and irrelevant details, there will be students developing illegitimate helps to get these just right on the exam.

TEACHING FOR THE TEST. An unwritten rule of teaching and testing is "Don't teach for the test." The basis for this is that students are supposed to learn a wide range of things in a class, and then the test is a random sample of these. How Jack does on the test is a good indication of how well Jack knows all of the things not asked. In the decade of the 1960's, however, we developed programmed learning, behavioral objectives and accountability. These embodied another ethic: the teacher and student should know exactly what is to be learned . . . learning activities should be designed to have this learning take place . . . evaluation should directly measure how well the intended learning has taken place. I have a class now that is based on ten behavioral objectives, and the students are told, the first day, that these are the basis for the final exam. The implications of this are critical because it directly challenges the dictum of not teaching for the test and suggests that learning should not be such a mysterious game.

Early in 1973, I wrote a letter to the chairman of my department discussing my philosophy of grading. I said:

> You have brought it to my attention that, in the name of accountability, you will be required to report the range and average of grades given by each departmental faculty member to the Dean. Presumably, this is relevant to someone's judgment that we do not give enough low grades . . . and that this result is somehow reprehensible. I certainly do not believe in giving grades carelessly and without designed evaluation, and therefore I present a brief thesis on my grading and how it relates to the learning process I attempt to direct in my class.

> The College of Education is the professional school concerned with preparing and improving the competence of teachers and other educators for the schools and communities of Illinois and other American states. It certainly should be cognizant of and willing to practice the best theory generated by the education profession. One of the most important themes, presently, is that the central task of education is to encourage learning—with the important riders that (1) the encouragement should extend beyond a particular class and (2) should be related to *actual* learning rather than merely to "getting a good grade."

> The philosophy behind a "normal curve" in grading is that about half of any class are going to exhibit what they have learned in a very ordinary or inferior way. Further, if A and B grades are valued more than C, D, and F grades, receiving a lower grade is supposed to motivate the learner to do better . . . the principle of punishment to get better performance. Also, there is a very individualistic, competitive ethic to this "traditional" grading system—there will be competition for the high grades, only half will succeed (so half will not succeed), and almost any helping of

one another is considered cheating. If the university is supposed to be, fundamentally, a "sorting" institution, one determining who shall *not* be able to achieve future goals, then grading on a curve and giving many low grades is perfectly proper.

Another potentially interesting observation: a "normal curve" of grades probably is easiest to achieve in a rather cold, "objective" classroom atmosphere, one strong with the odor of "there's more to learn than any of you can—if you learn, okay . . . if not, who cares." When everything done by students is translated into numbers (often fairly arbitrarily, originally) and then these numbers are interpreted as reality, it is much easier to give a C and then say, "you were 2 points from a B . . . there's nothing I can (or want to) do about it."

My philosophy, however, is that this university (or at least *my* classes) should be primarily an institution of learning. I also am more convinced that rewards bring forth more learning—now and in the future beyond the classroom—than do punishments. (And, practically speaking for future teachers, since pay scales typically are related to graduate credits and degrees earned and since the attempt to earn these is related to grades previously received, C's, D's and F's are forms of punishment. As I perceive the various professions within education, I see that an individual practitioner rarely has to display what he knows or can do in the form of answers to a test (particularly multiple choice or true-false). Therefore, if the evaluation of learning takes some of the many forms that are more similar to those learners will have to meet in a teaching life, it tends to be more realistic.

In my experience, particularly over the last five years, the more truly different, but relevant, forms of evaluation that are utilized, the more difficult it is for me to come up with a normal curve of grades. With a wide variety of ways available and required, the majority of learners find ways to express what they have learned *with performance beyond the average and ordinary*. The converse, I believe, is also true. The simplest way to establish a "normal" distribution of grades is to give only one kind of evaluation, so that those who succeed are rewarded and those who do not are reinforced in their perceptions of themselves as average or below average learners. Further, if no relearning is allowed, then the ones who learn something correctly and completely the first time are rewarded, and those who must take a time or so more are not.

If our concern in the public schools is that children and youth learn, however many attempts it takes, do we increase or decrease the possibility of new teachers being sensitive to this need if all *they* have experienced in teacher education is the competitive, "strong shall survive" style of evaluation?

In addition to a variety of ways of being evaluated, students in my classes often have chances to relearn an idea or a concept and express it correctly and with excellence without penalty for not having done so the first time. In other classes, particularly summer workshops, I use a form of contract system where students can determine if they are willing to do what is necessary for an A or a B, or whether they are satisfied in doing the work for a C or a D.

I return unsatisfactory work quickly with suggestions for change or modification. In this system where the individual is competing with himself and some standard of excellence developed jointly by her/him and me, I find the number of average or below performers to be "fewer than would be expected."

I never have consciously used a grade as a punishment. I reserve the right, however, as a participant in academic freedom and as a responsible senior professional in the education field, to *occasionally* use a grade as an encouragement—to give a grade higher than a student objectively deserves in order to encourage him or her to continue in the field.

In short, virtually everything I do in a classroom is intended to stimulate learning. In this regard, I am an avid, perhaps close to a fanatic, professional. (I regard guiding and encouraging in the learning process essentially as a seduction process, which is to be preferred to rape, [which is a better analogy for much traditional education]. In my view, seduction is much more enjoyable, for all concerned parties, than rape.) I evaluate in a variety of ways; return tests, papers and projects promptly, often with extensive written comments, criticisms and suggestions; I allow "second chances" to indicate learning, with little or no penalty; I use contracts to encourage each student to do her/his best . . . and when "one's best" is really encouraged, it is surprising how many edge up "above average."

I try to create a warm atmosphere of comfortable learning in the classroom. I encourage much more the notion that it is important to learn from one another than one of keeping what one knows inviolately personal.

I do not give many "low" grades, because at the end of a course, I typically find very few students who have not learned and cannot express it with excellence. I also have very few who say or seem to feel, "Well, I'm glad that's over . . . I hope I never have to take another course . . . from him . . . or in that area."

However, it also is important to note that I have high standards, particularly in relation to participating in the learning process. Some students truly earn C's, D's, and F's, and when they do, they receive them. But I work hard to see that no more get such grades than really desire such, usually by vivid displays of lethargy and lassitude.

One final comment relative to the profession and discipline of health education. It is a discipline in which the essential skills are communication and motivation, and its skillful practice can potentially help many other human beings to live more full and functional lives. Communication with and motivation of a number of "segments" of the total U.S. population is often accomplished best by "educators" who do not do well in traditional forms of academic evaluation. In order to educate these needed professionals we must develop evaluation forms that relate more to what they will actually do and less to traditional forms. In this sense, we can encourage professional excellence only by redefining academic excellence . . . which may well include looking for the ways in which learners *are* excellent rather than merely measuring how they are not by limited, traditional evaluation modes.

In conclusion, I grade conscientiously. I find relatively few learners who do not learn with some marked excellence, and I am less and less worried that I do not have "normal curves."

Should I be . . . really?

THE FUNDAMENTAL EVALUATION IN HEALTH EDUCATION IS APPLICATION. Can the learner apply what has been learned accurately and appropriately, in a variety of situations? Can she/he apply both content and process appropriately? That is, does she/he know how to find information she/he has forgotten or never known, quickly and efficiently? And one of the most important forms of application is . . . how effectively can she/he communicate health ideas to others and motivate them to consider what might be a healthier way? In other words, the ultimate evaluation of health learning for Sam and Sally is (a) how healthy each is . . . how well each functions . . . throughout the many unpredictable situations of life and (b) how effective as a health educator each is with family, friends, and others in life situations. You live it . . . and you also give it away.

Health education is never going to be perfect. It's another game we play in which we want to achieve more than is possible. Evaluation makes it clearer what has been accomplished. And also what has not been accomplished. Each year there is even more to learn than the year before, with issues often becoming more complex rather than simpler. There also are more ways to learn. Example: Electronic information systems of the future will provide much up-to-date knowledge, but the citizen will have to be able to make the darn things work.

Technically for school health instruction, evaluation is that portion of the curriculum that indicates how well learners have achieved the stated objectives. But also, evaluation should tell us what else has happened that may lead to new objectives, fresh learning approaches, revised content, and new and more vital resource materials. And then these, as aids to learning, would be evaluated . . . and, again, what else happened. And so it goes.

SUMMARY.

- The two purposes of evaluation are to:
    - (1) assess to what extent what was intended was accomplished
    - (2) assess what else happened . . . what other things were learned
- Health education is both content and process, and therefore how well students have learned how to learn also should be evaluated.

- Evaluation of classroom behavior is much simpler than of outside-of-school personal behavior.
- At present the main thrust of evaluation of school learning is on the basis of learners being individualistic and competitive.
- Some forms of evaluation are designed to be learning experiences in themselves; some are not.
- There are advantages and disadvantages to both objective and subjective styles of evaluation.
- The more different forms of evaluation employed, the less likely a teacher is to have a normal curve of grades for a class.
- One philosophy of evaluation assumes a certain number will do poorly and the form is designed to accurately discover which students these are; another assumes that all should learn certain things and that teaching for the test is legitimate.

Chapter XV

Health Education
Beyond the School

This book is presented under the banner of the Joint Committee on Health Problems in Education of the National Education Association and the American Medical Association, and is therefore mostly about health education in schools. However, an earlier chapter presented the premise that health education occurs in many different settings and throughout the whole of life. Health education does come from learning under a knowledgeable, professional teacher, but it also comes out of interaction with other people in life situations, from self-directed learning experiences, and from trying to teach other people. It runs the range from very formal to very informal. It also runs the gamut from that of which the learner is very conscious to that of which he is virtually unconscious. One more gamut, that from the very accurate to the very inaccurate, silly, or downright dangerous. We have to allow for all sorts of consistent and inconsistent messages.

THE FAMILY. Let us begin with the family, an arena for a total range of health education.

"Ralph, you've been pushing yourself too hard . . . stay home today, rest in bed, eat the special things I fix for you, and you'll avoid getting sick like you have before."

"Jenny, maybe that medication is good for your physical ills, but it seems to be ruining your disposition . . . you'd better go back to the doctor."

Husband and wife, interacting closely, are almost certain to offer each other diagnostic reactions and helpful information. As indicated earlier, one of the purposes of school health education is to help learners become better potential health educators, non-professional style. This capacity is probably developed best with intimate friends, and the marriage relationship is one of the most likely. When marriages are good, the health education between partners tends to be lovingly given and received and is a strengthening factor. However, what one partner intends as a helpful health message may be interpreted as nagging by the other. As marriage relationships go sour, this tendency increases and may become a visible factor in marriage break-up. In other words, the nature of a health-related communication may reflect the quality of the relationship between the marriage partners. The words:

> Dan, I really think you're trying to do too much . . . you're not sleeping well, you're irritable . . . you're just not functioning normally . . . and I'm worried . . .

come out one way when the wife loves and is genuinely concerned about Dan . . . and another way when her concern is that Dan might die and leave her to her own resources . . . or worse, that he might become incapacitated and become a burden on her.

Put in terms of the broadened definition of health developed early in this tome, the relationship of a couple is determined by the mental, emotional and spiritual health of each, and this social dimension of health then greatly affects the quality of health education between them.

PARENT-CHILD INTERCHANGES. Some pattern of communication has been established, then, by the time a child arrives to enlarge the family, both in size and in range of years. One of the fundamental responsibilities of parents is health education of their child or children. Many early first communications, verbal and otherwise, have a health component. Parents are concerned that a child grow and develop normally. Much of this concern results in a lot of safety education. Modern life is full of hazards, and until a youngster can understand how to adapt to the devices, chemicals, nature phenomena (fire, water, air, earth), and other living things inhabiting his ecosystem, parents must warn, watch and protect . . . in order that the babe might survive to understand.

Yet, safety education may contain more implications than intended. Our first two sons were about sixteen months apart in age. By the time the second one was six months or so and crawling around, the older was still less than two and wanted to play with his baby brother. We judged that there was some danger to Mike from being dragged around, etc., but also that excessive admonitions might create negative feelings in Bob. So we kept these to a minimum and banked on the toughness of the toy to survive being played with.

A major challenge of parental health education is knowing when and how to change from commands and admonitions to more truly educational experiences, wherein the youngster understands why certain behaviors and non-behaviors are considered more desirable than others. Another is knowing when to let a child learn from an experience, when to try to have her/him experience it vicariously and decide on the basis of potentialities and probabilities. How long do parents say:

> Eat your vegetables!
>
> Put on your sweater!
>
> Brush and floss your teeth!
>
> I don't want you associating with those kids!

Stop being so selfish!

You are not allowed to smoke!

And when, and under what circumstances do they begin to let their progeny assess the values and demerits of the behaviors for themselves? In many cases, of course, the youngster feels that this should happen before the parents can comfortably go this route.

If parents persist in restricting the child sometime after she/he feels a desire for independence, there may be some clashes, but the child may also perceive this concern as an evidence of love and gain from it feelings of security. Conversely, if parents give in too quickly to the child's demands, this may be perceived as lack of love and generate feelings of insecurity . . . they really don't care about me. Yet, independence has to develop, and hence the game goes on, sometimes played with skill and sometimes with abominable ineptness. In contrast to many other games, of course, if this one is played well by all involved, everyone wins.

NON-PARENT ADULTS. "All involved" introduces another element into family health education. Adults other than parents may be closely enough associated with a youngster to be helpful in the education process. Grandparents, aunts, uncles, friends of the family, or neighbors may, in certain circumstances, give information, communicate attitudes and become involved in a child's growing and learning. Obviously, these associations can be of variable quality.

One of the chronic reluctances about school health education stems from the fear that school is trying to usurp the prerogatives of the home and family. One of the persistent arguments for health education in school, on the other hand, is that certain youngsters get a set of pretty sad lessons at home and are entitled to some means to rebut these potentially harmful learnings.

ESPECIALLY HELPFUL . . . SEX EDUCATION. One of the times in which these non-parental adults can be most helpful is in what could be generically called sex education, which deals with developing into a sexual being and relating to other sexual beings. Many parents can be adequate to excellent in telling their offspring about reproduction ("See the little kitty being born . . .") while the child is still a child. But, after the progeny pass puberty, the circumstances change. Now the sexual relations to discuss are between human beings rather than guppies and groundhogs.

The relationships are complex . . . feelings are partly conscious and partly unconscious . . . different between parent and child of the same sex and of the opposite sex. . . . In short, there may be enough apprehensiveness and discomfort about what portions of questions and answers are theory and what are practice to prevent the sexual education session from becoming a reality. The non-parental adult has consequent opportunities to answer and ask questions of the youngsters, unencumbered by the various conflicts of parent, husband/wife.

SIBLINGS. Other potentially major health-related interchanges within the family are between and among siblings. The only child misses this opportunity . . . and, of course, having siblings is no guarantee that there will be any helpful relations. However, siblings have had certain common experiences as well as their own individual ones. Opportunities for communication are many, and learning from these closest of relatives can be invaluable. Some years ago, while teaching "Marriage and Family," I received a paper from a student that was entitled "I Had Six Parents." The girl was born when her youngest sibling was sixteen years old. So the paper described ways in which her siblings, particularly the sisters, had helped her grow up. She saw it all as a unique and wonderful experience . . . that she had been particularly fortunate.

HEALTH EDUCATION: HOME AND/OR SCHOOL. Okay, let's say it again . . . some folks perceive the school and the home as competing with each other in regard to some health issues. Totally abstinent parents may be afraid that their children are being taught that it's all right to drink in school. Many parents might worry that the issue of abortion is being taught in school when they think it should not be.

A chiropractor or a health food operator, as parents, might be upset with possible aspersions on their contribution to health . . . and therefore on their self-worth as parents.

On the other hand, society can justifiably feel that parents do not have unlimited right to miseducate their offspring, since the latter will be relatively independent citizens of the society much longer than they will be dependent children.

In a mobile and multi-valued society, do the schools have a responsibility for broadening a youngster's perception of how life can be lived? How does this stand up against parents' rights to raise children as they believe?

To the extent that it is not clearly settled, health education will be in the school curriculum . . . but some of it will frequently be controversial. For many children and youth, the school health program should be seen as complementary and supplementary to that of the home. For others, it is a new window through which to view healthy functioning in different and positive ways. It is anyone's guess and value judgment what the relative proportions should be.

RELIGION. For many people, religion is an agency of health education in some important areas. Religion implies a community of similarly believing folk meeting together, sharing values, and agreeing that it is important to bring up children in the right way.

Probably the most positive health education is that of encouraging an individual to be less selfish and consider the welfare of others at least equal to that of self.

HEALTH AGENCIES: TYPES. Some variety of agencies within any community have responsibilities that include health education. One way to sort these is:

- tax-supported agencies (mainly public health departments)
- non-tax supported (commercial, professional and voluntary agencies)

Another classification would be:

- those concerned mostly with education toward primary prevention
- those concerned with education relating to treatment, rehabilitation, and secondary and tertiary prevention

How about one more?

- those concerned with a general range of health-related issues
- those concerned with a very specific issue (cancer, multiple sclerosis, family planning, environmental preservation . . .)

THREE EDUCATIONAL APPROACHES. In some instances, the education is carried on by trained health educators; in other cases, it is done by other health personnel, like physicians, dentists, nurses, sanitarians, program administrators, secretaries, clerks, aides. . . . The approaches tend to be of a similar range as that described for school classrooms. Consider an all-day conference on smoking sponsored by the American Lung Association, the American Heart Association, the Cancer Society, and the City Health Department. The first speaker makes a very factual presentation, composed of facts, figures, charts, graphs, and extrapolations. The speaker was selected from the Speaker's Bureau of the Lung Association. It was supposed to be a middle-aged internist, but at the last minute he cancelled, and so it was done by a young assistant professor of biology at the university. It could have been given by any of a dozen speakers, and it would have been about the same. The second morning feature was a presentation by a well-known film actor, who, having recovered from lung cancer, had a very dramatic story to tell. It was personal, gripping and intended to make young people feel the fear, uncertainty, and helplessness of this result of smoking. In the afternoon, a skillful health educator arranged the audience into working groups of eight and really got them interacting over the motivations for and against smoking as a teenager. Each group role-played some original situations, trying to become more conscious of and comfortable with ways of keeping from smoking . . . or at least of preventing the development of habitual smoking. The youths applied knowledge, acted out situations, reacted to one another, and made some commitments. The health educator simply had the plan organized and helped it to happen.

The three general approaches to education, then, are (1) authoritative, factual telling, (2) charismatic, personal relating, and (3) active involvement of people in the learning process.

AUTHORITATIVE TELLERS . . . WHY? Physicians, dentists, nurses, and allied health personnel tend to be authoritative tellers when they act as educators. Possible reasons for this are several:

"I have the information they need . . . the simplest and easiest approach is to tell them . . . I am the authority . . . I know."

"Education is only a small part of what I do . . . and I'm better trained to do the other . . . so I want to get my educational responsibilities accomplished as quickly as possible."

"Frankly, I'm not at all sure how to use some of these educational techniques . . . basically what I've experienced in education is being told by an authority, so I tend to do the same."

"I certainly learned all right from authoritative lectures. It's a matter of concentration. If people really want to learn, they can."

SYMBOLIC VALUE. This is not an attempt to put down other health professionals. All of these reasons have merit, and for people who have some knowledge of the medical terminology and a desire to learn, a physician's presentation can be quite educational. And it may be helpful in other ways, too. In *Mirage of Health,* Dubos describes the symbol of the physician in England just before the triumph of experimental science over clinical art as the gold-headed cane. Of it he says,

> . . . the skill symbolized by the gold-headed cane was not mere charlatanism. It grew in no small part from the physician's awareness—even though ill defined and often subconscious—of the many factors which play a part in the causation and manifestations of disease.[1]

We have had experimental science for 150 years, but, even in the minds of many patients today, the image of the physician with the authority of the gold-headed cane is a comforting one. An anthropological study of medical care and health education in a Chilean clinic[2] disclosed that patients listened attentively to the doctor's instructions, appeared to understand, but actually had little or no idea of what he had said. Part of the difficulty was vocabulary, but another part was that they didn't consider it appropriate to understand the doctor. It was an honor to be addressed by him, and one gloried in that. To understand what to

---

[1] Dubos, Rene, *Mirage of Health,* pg. 123. By permission of Harper & Row.

[2] Simmons, Ozzie G., "The Clinical Team in A Chilean Health Center," Case 12 in Paul, Benjamin (Ed.), *Health, Culture and Community.* New York: Russell Sage Foundation, 1955. pp. 339-340.

do, one listened to and learned from the nurse. Undoubtedly, American patients are more advanced than Chilean peasants of 30 years ago, but I doubt that many patients have advanced very far from this respect for authority. Experimental science has not made medicine a cut-and-dried set of techniques; there is still some mystery; some live and some die. So the authoritative lecture may communicate a basis for confidence— that may be as important as the statistics, the syndromes and the sequelae.

SINGLE ISSUE AGENCIES . . . DIFFICULT. The earlier categorizations let you in on the fact that some agencies are concerned with a single issue and can therefore concentrate their efforts on fund-raising for monies to research, serve and educate about the particular issue. Examples of single issue health agencies are the American Heart Association, the American Cancer Society and the American Lung Association, all with regional, state and some local affiliates. It seems to be increasingly difficult, however, for these agencies to concentrate. The Heart people want to reduce, even conquer heart disease, but this gets them into exercise, diet, strep infections, smoking and heredity. Heart and Cancer and Lung Associations thus join together in opposing smoking. The Cancer Society is interested because it probably does cause cancers of the lung, pharynx, lip and other areas of the body. The American Lung Association's interest stems from a concern for the reduction of emphysema and other respiratory diseases. The Heart Association is concerned because of the proven relationship between smoking and a variety of circulatory ailments.

These three organizations are joined by 29 other organizations in the National Interagency Council on Smoking (NIC). Nevertheless, it must be noted that even with all this united effort behind a particular non-behavior (not smoking), in 1974 the downward trend in smoking has been reversed, mainly due to the rapid increase in smoking by women.

HEALTH DEPARTMENTS . . . WIDE RANGE. The fundamental point is that, despite desires to concentrate on particular health issues, human beings will not cooperate and consistently have only a particular malady. Hence, health departments have a more all-purpose orientation. They are less troubled with overlapping conditions, but many have difficulty in determining which diseases or ill-health conditions are the most proper for public funds. Public health departments traditionally have had just concerns for improving conditions that individual citizens, however conscientious, simply could not deal with adequately, such as sanitation and safety of food, milk and water.

Almost parallel concerns have been for protecting the community from disease, particularly through immunization programs. With this service, they overlap into the domain of private medicine. This is usually resolved by a recognition of the fact that both are concerned with the health of the community. Although there may be public and private misunderstandings in some communities, there is increasing cooperation between private and community medicine.

SELF-HELP GROUPS. An increasingly important educational force in communities, particularly significant in really changing behavior, are various problem-oriented self-help groups. The original prototype seems to have been Alcoholics Anonymous, started by two chronic drunks back in the 1930's who got together in desperation and promised to try to keep each other sober. It worked, and the movement began . . . and has spawned others in more recent years. The characteristics of such groups are:

- All members have basically the same problem (drink too much, are too fat, gamble compulsively, take drugs, are divorced).
- Members honestly admit that they have the problem and accept the admissions and comradeship of others with the same problem.
- Members help one another to overcome the problem, encouraging one another and rewarding one another's successes in developing a life-style without the problem.

With obesity being related casually to many fatal and debilitating conditions and with American culture dedicated to over-eating and to underexercising, the addition of unwanted pounds has become fairly endemic. Many groups, such as TOPS (Take Off Pounds Sensibly), have aided persons in healthful weight control. A recent and particularly successful group is Weight Watchers. Obese people meet together regularly, admit they need to and want to lose weight and keep it off, weigh before the group and receive applause for weight lost. They tell each other how they are able to stay on the diet prescribed. The education is essentially personal. It appears to be the participative process that tends to produce the healthful results.

THERAPY GROUPS. The last decade has seen the growth of a wide range of therapy, encounter and relating groups. The main value comes out of the process of members relating to one another, sharing ideas and concerns, and establishing genuine feelings of belonging. The presence and the high quality of professional leadership is important. With poor quality or no professional leadership, the presence of one or more really sick people in a group can have serious consequences. The competent, skillfull leader actually abets the group process and, further, is there to deal with the unexpected emergencies that can arise out of the interactions.

TELEVISION . . . AND RADIO. "And now CBS presents a special documentary. . . ."

"Tonight's show centers on an athlete who is taking dope to mask symptoms of illness in order to complete the basketball season."

"Fast, fast, fast relief . . . Doctors recommend . . . Tests in a famous laboratory prove. . . ."

Yes, offerings on television and, to some extent, radio are part of community health education—positive and negative. Documentary and news programs can present factual information and yet have an eye-catching, compelling quality to them as well. Dramatic programs and movies certainly deal with many kinds of emotional conflicts and decision-making situations and with virtually all styles and phases of marriage and family life. Medically-oriented programs deal with simple to very complex health problems, their treatment, cure, and prevention. No one really knows how much useful information comes from television programs of all types . . . but there is undoubtedly a great deal of misinformation.

Commercials give information on conditions and products. Various governmental agencies regulate commercials so that no blatant untruths are presented. The main area of exaggeration and half-truth is in relation to the relative value of two competing brands of essentially the same product—(toothpaste, aspirin, laxatives, vitamins . . .). Part of successful adaptation as a modern American (which must be accomplished early in life) is to develop a high tolerance for commercials and advertisements. Obviously these have some influence, but ardent affluent television watchers and radio listeners soon recognize that they actually consider purchasing only a small portion of what is advertised and actually come home with a small part of this small portion. However compelling and unique a commercial may be, it is useful only for a short time. Part of the education of commercials, then, by their very profusion, is that "you don't take most of them seriously."

OTHER MEDIA. Billboards, newspapers, magazines, giveaways, leaflets, junk mail, mail catalogues, and promotions for a number of causes present health education in myriad forms and voices. A leaflet for a missionary program may give information on malnutrition and attempts to counter it in Latin America. A health insurance flyer may give facts on costs of hospitalization. A newspaper carries an interview with a woman who survived after a plane crash in the mountains, presenting some provocative ideas about survival with one's own resources. Books and journals obviously are part of the educational scene. All of these compete for attention. Even an avid reader finds she/he can read less and less of what there is potentially to read. How to discriminate in this culture of impossible cultures is one of the learning processes that must be mastered. Why? Because an unfortunate response of frustration over choices is to withdraw and read almost nothing . . . a sad choice in today's world . . . but, still an understandable one.

HEALTH EDUCATION IN OTHER SETTINGS. An individual educated in health education finds her/himself participating in many arenas. Some of these are school-community related, patient-related in hospitals and physicians' offices, industry-related and government-related.

A SUMMARY

- Health education occurs first and continuously in one's immediate family—between marriage partners, parents and children, other adults and other children, and among siblings.
- Religion, for some people, has health education components. For these people, health education is related to religious beliefs.
- Many health professionals, with important information, use authoritative telling as their main educational technique.
- Self-help and therapy groups often combine education about others and their perceptions of life with education about self.
- The mass media, among other functions, allows for incidental education about many health-related issues.
- A professional health educator can function in many settings.
- In the future, there should be less difference between the styles of health education most effective in the school and community.
- If health education in schools can help prepare young people for the continuing process of learning that will continue in the community and that will carry over after schooltime, it will be accomplishing a potentially worthy goal.
- In the better school health education programs, students will be directed in learning experiences that offer them opportunity to learn some things from the community . . . and in the process, the community learns some things from them.
- School . . . Community. They complement each other. Each can accomplish its goals best through cooperation with the other.

Chapter XVI

Some Future
for
Health Education

There will be plenty of health education in the future. In one form or another, people will advise each other about ways to play life's games that are better . . . more rewarding . . . less punishing . . . than others. There undoubtedly will be some institutionalized health education, too . . . in schools, through community agencies, in physicians' and dentists' offices, in hospitals, and in health maintenance and delivery facilities. There certainly will be health education in some new, as yet unimagined, arenas of human interaction. Wherever and however it occurs, health education predictably will continue to be:

- accurate and inaccurate

Part of this accuracy question will be due to inadequacies in the educator, part due to wrong perceptions or interpretations by learners, and part due to the fact that authorities do not agree, so that to be accurate according to one will guarantee inaccuracy according to another. The troublesome thing about inaccuracy is that it can be communicated to others with the same zeal and persuasiveness as accuracy.

Most messages in the future seem destined to be incomplete, because more and more will be known about every health issue. It is possible that some new knowledge will pull together many of today's fragments, producing a simpler and more complete description of a total health area. This is possible, but improbable, given the various dimensions of health issues.

CONSERVATIVE AND RADICAL (two interpretations by the author). One interpretation of these ends of a continuum (rather than dichotomy) is that conservative means "doing things the way I've been doing them," and radical means "doing things in new and different ways." Some health education will encourage doing something "like my mother did," "like I learned in medical school," "the way we all do it in this commune." Other health education, by process as much as by content, will urge trying new approaches, rejecting the tried and true almost as a matter of principle.

Another interpretation of these terms has "conservative" meaning "safe" . . . not taking chances, while radical encompasses the opposite . . . various forms of risk-taking behavior. As has been said before, traditional health education typically opts for safety and few chances.

The future, however, will contain numerous opportunities to take a risk for some good reason.

AN INTERESTING CASE IN POINT is a person choosing to have her/himself frozen before death in order to await a cure for some current malady. Let's say it is Genevieve A., a prototype of a small number already cryonically resting. Genevieve has a confirmed diagnosis of a form of cancer that typically will spread rapidly and soon be fatal. One of her medical consultants predicts that an effective cure will be available for this in a few years. If she were to be quickly frozen now, before the cancer has progressed too far and then returned to life after the cure has been perfected and is available, she might have many more healthy years. If she is conservative and will not take the chance, she probably will die. If she takes the risk, there is probably no way to know if it has been a healthy or unhealthy choice until the attempt is made to return her to life. If she waits too long to make the choice, she reduces her chance of survival even if the freezing-thawing process is successful. If she decides too soon, and the process fails, it amounts to some combination of murder and suicide. Okay, this seems far-out, but each new possibility for better health or longer life will have to be tried out with some person, then another and others. There was a first heart transplant . . . and then more. There will be more firsts, all with automatic risks. But, "be safe and die" seem anachronistic, too.

OTHER PREDICTIONS ABOUT HEALTH EDUCATION: GENERAL EDUCATION. Health education could have an important, lasting place in the school curriculum if we, the culture, should come to see this as a significant new arena for general human understanding—comparable to present feelings about English literature, biological science, history, Spanish. . . . Though each of these has certain practical applications, they are in the curriculum as aspects of general education, not as means to solve certain problems. If students do not speak and read Spanish very well, or appreciate Spanish culture at the end of a class, the twin solutions are: improve teaching-learning or study for another year. The judgment if the students don't learn, to do away with the course, does not seem appropriate for these general education courses. In the future, as the culture reforms its perceptions for learning, health education may become one of those important general education courses.

PROBLEM-SOLVING. Another basis for improvement would be the future view that the schools are a really important part of the problem-solving process for persons and safety. In this view, a major focus of the schools' curricula would be courses and experiences that deal with human, group and social problems. Health education would be big,

dealing with problems as they begin to arise in community consciousness . . . like education about physical fitness in the 1940's, sex education (in some places) in the 1960's, drug education in the early 1970's
. . . and, perhaps education about venereal disease and nutrition in
the 1970's.

"But wait," you undoubtedly are saying, "surely health education
will be seen as a part of the solution when a problem is fairly full
blown." That certainly is logical, and it is a possibility as we move
through the next decades. However, the danger is that the schools will
have to keep balancing their eclectic responsibilities about as they do
now. Health education is not as important a part of general education
as it should be for primary prevention. Health education is screamed
for when there is a perceived problem and then neglected when the
problem diminishes in relation to new, more seemingly critical ones.

COMMUNITY PRIORITY? Health education in the community,
through various non-school agencies, could become more important,
but its impact on youth would depend on the community's relative
concern for the young . . . in competition with other age groups. There
are relatively fewer children and youth each year, and relatively more
of the elderly. The priorities thus could shift in the direction of:

PRIORITIES

Middle-aged. This segment is increasing in proportion . . . is the
main producing, earning, and taxpaying group . . . is becoming
more motivated toward healthful living . . . expensive treatments
can be prevented or postponed if health education takes.

Elderly. This segment is increasing . . . is the most conscious of
health and the most motivated to avoid ill-health . . . increasingly
demanding of education programs . . . have time to participate.

Children and Youth. This segment is decreasing . . . is the healthiest, the least conscious of health, the least interested in health
education . . . should be a higher priority, but the other priorities
seem more insistent.

Health education in conjunction with actual medical care facilities—hospitals, clinics, health maintenance organizations—seems to be
developing. It seems increasingly wasteful not to take advantage of both
the motivations toward better health and the time patients have (waiting
for treatment or as in-patients) and offer such folk some educational
experiences. The major breakthrough would be the inclusion of pay-
ment for education (as part of preventive care) as a benefit under health
insurance. Organization could take many forms, but the psychological
counseling model—some individual, some family, some in groups of
varying sizes—probably would be a sound take-off point.

FUTURE I AND II. In considering the future, let us turn now to a more basic choice of direction for the culture. Perhaps there are more than two directions, but as I have ruminated on future possibilities in a naturalistic frame of reference I find it most productive to think of two basic orientations. (Considering the supernatural provides several other directions, which will be eschewed here.)

- Future I involves the logical continuation of the ideal American life-style, which takes us farther away from the majority of other human beings inhabiting the earth at this time.
- Future II involves consciously trying to move closer to the rest of mankind . . . to reduce the distance and keep it as small as possible.

In Future I, we would continue, even expand, our aspirations for better and longer lives for everyone. To achieve more longevity, we would expend more effort and funds on cures and non-behavioral preventions* of heart and circulatory system diseases and various forms of cancer. Fashioning a better life would entail more use of non-muscle power, most of it produced from fossil fuels for the foreseeable future (but, eventually, some more abundant and cheaper fuel). This would mean more air conditioning and central heating, more cars, planes, trucks, and railroads . . . more automation, meaning more leisure and less work for U.S. citizens. Controls on pollution and recycling would be present and functional, but would require even more fuel and non-muscle energy. Though population control would be generally accepted, the population would continue to expand, due to longer life and immigration, rather than births. The average age of the population would rise steadily, the influence of youth would diminish, and conservative attitudes would tend to prevail. Because of a larger population, there would be pressures for more control of individual deviance and more homogeneity. All of this, of course, would be for our own good, for our happiness.

Part of the responsibility of being a human being is to foresee possible side effects of progress, judge how likely they are to be, and make those hard choices that involve, Is it worth the risk? Sometimes staying healthy involves taking risks.

Finally, the gap between the U.S. and most of the rest of humankind would grow larger, and the response from at least some of these would be as to the selfish rich kid.

In Future II, the major emphasis would be on coming closer to, or at least not going too far beyond, the rest of humankind. This would involve reduced use of resources and therefore lessened pollution and waste. In general, the ethic would be that humankind wins, ultimately, only when it suffers its share of losses. Birth control would be improved

---

* Preventions that would not entail changing present harmful styles of living.

in order to eliminate, insofar as possible, unwanted children. No other restrictions on having children would be instituted; instead a more natural, ecological view of death would be encouraged, with no special procedures for prolonging life after age 65 or 70. Those that survived to old age would do so basically with their own resources instead of costly medical-technological ones. Average age of the population would be somewhere in the 30-35 range.

The American diet would shift toward less meat and more grains and vegetables. Priorities for uses of non-muscle power would be set from the top down and bottom up. Top priority would be th' preservation of food, and low would be large advertising displays and the manufacture of luxury or novelty items. We would have less central heat and central air conditioning and therefore a bit more seasonal discomfort. Electrical power might even be allotted to geographic areas, an indirect way to affect the redistribution of population. The culture would value the re-use of containers and the recycling of glass, metal, garbage, paper, etc. Nothing would be seen as a waste, but only as a potential resource. Transportation would have as its dominant values less power and speed, less pollution and more efficiency. Two and four cylinder vehicles, checked for efficiency twice yearly would be normative. Transportation in central cities (down to cities 25,000-30,000) would be limited to walking, bicycling, public transportation and electric car. Airline schedules would disappoint some, but would insure maximally full planes to justify the tremendous gulping of fuel. A lessened manufacturing of products would mean more services and, gradually, more muscle power.

The size of population is absolutely crucial in Future I, because a growing population attempting to universally implement and improve the American standard of living would consume non-renewable resources in devastating ways. In Future II population is not as critical as the general effect of the dominant life-style on the environment. If the population is relatively stable, a good balance is easier to achieve; if it is not stable, there is still more life ahead. If we develop new, practical, non-harmfully polluting sources of energy (solar, wind, ocean currents, fusion, fission. . . .), then we in Future II might more justifiably move back toward Future I. Yet, if we had become hooked on sharing with the rest of humankind, we might not want to.

HUXLEY AS FUTURIST. For those readers who are Huxley buffs, the preceding may seem to have some relationship to two novels by him, *Brave New World*[1] and *Island.*[2] *Brave New World,* chronicling life in

---

[1] Huxley, Aldous, *Brave New World*. New York: Harper & Row, Bantam Books, 1932, 1966. 177 pp.

[2] Huxley, Aldous, *Island*. New York: Harper & Row, Bantam Books, 1962. 295 pp.

the Society of Our Ford, is the obvious triumph of a naturalistic-scientific-technological way of life designed to make and keep people happy and satisfied. In the emotional climax, the protagonist is pushed to self-destruction because he questions some of the established values of the culture. One obvious point of difference between this and Future I is that in *Brave New World* each citizen was taught early in life to accept, as a fair exchange, a life of full, undiseased vigor for a certain death somewhere in the sixth decade of life. In contrast, and in more contiguity with Future II, Huxley's last novel, *Island,* told of a culture developed scientifically, but in harmony with the environment and the rest of life. Muscle power was valued, because scientific findings showed physical work was necessary to well-being. The culture adapted to individual desires and the development of individuals—it had freedom—but it did so by limiting births and letting deaths occur naturally.

One major generalization from both of these Futures and novels is that freedom to be different, individually and in life-style, is directly dependent on a non-expanding population. If population continues to increase, under either Future, there would appear to be more regulation and less tolerance for deviating from the societal norm. Obviously, if one agrees with the norm, there is no hassle. If one does not, life will not appear to be good as it might.

If the two novels do have some similarity to the two Futures, they suggest different directions for the advance of civilization. One civilization is based on more and better technology; the other is based on more aware social and personal relationships. Perhaps there is some perfect synthesis in between, and the anthropological evidence certainly affirms that the advance of civilization has no necessary relation to more technology or even longer life.

TOLERANCE FOR DIFFERENCE. Less tolerance for deviating from the societal norm—did you just read this phrase as descriptive of our probable future? Just to becloud the prognosis, it could be argued, from using the present as a starting point, that the future will be marked by more acceptance as normal of people whose behavior or life-style was once clearly called deviant from the societal norms. As a wider range of anything emerges, styles of clothing, sexual practices, language forms, religious, intimate relationships—the original norm—tend to become less compelling. For this to remain as a condition of the future, there would need to develop a genuine tolerance for differences that has yet to be seen in any culture. The alternative could be a fractionated culture where differences are evident but where people with them relate to each other as little as possible. In an earlier discussion of behavior modification it was noted that the opposite of rewarding was seen to be ignoring rather than punishing. Perhaps the societal analogue is that if certain groups cannot really punish others for not doing what is right, they can jolly well ignore them. More freedom is purchased at this price: less relating, less cohesiveness and more diversity.

HEALTHY? This could be a healthy society with opportunities for everyone to do her/his own thing. An earlier chapter dealt with ecological perspective; this suggests that those who are good personal and social adapters naturally prefer this kind of society and thrive on it. Those who do not adapt so well are uncomfortable in it and balance between (1) surviving with some supportive counselling, (2) organizing and trying to bring society back where it should be, and (3) slumping into apathetic existence.

FUTURE SHOCK. Part of the above concept obviously relates to Toffler's notion of *Future Shock*.[3] This most menacing malady is a catchy name for a total personality's inability, finally, to deal with a present that is too unlike the future she/he had envisioned. The condition has a range of symptoms, from hyperaggressiveness to self-destructive apathy, but two characteristic ones are anxiety and indecisiveness. A somewhat extreme example I developed for a recent class:

> Oscar has just lost his job with the university because tenure has been repealed. He also just has discovered that his 70-year-old mother smokes grass, that his wife has signed up to have her body frozen shortly before death, that his daughter is studying to be an acupuncturist, and that his son is a homosexual, announcing his coming marriage to his boyfriend.

One by one, Oscar might have been able to deal with these changes in the social security that he had come to depend on. He might have been able to deal with a blow to the stereotype about mothers' behaviors and what ages do what . . . with challenges to his assumptions about death, about a proper occupation for his daughter and about legitimate medical care . . . and with an affront to his values and perceptions about right sexual relations and proper marriage. All together they shock him into a state of dysfunction.

WIDER ACCEPTANCE OF HEALTH CARE PRACTICES? Predictably, too, with this more accepting future, the counselling help that Oscar might seek would be less regulated and predictable. Osteopaths generally have been accepted as legitimate medical practitioners in an almost unlimited way. Some insurance policies now pay for chiropractic treatment regardless of its scientifically unproven status according to the value, "If it's what the patient wants. . . ." Nurse practitioners now assume responsibilities for actions and decisions that would have

---

[3] Toffler, Alvin, *Future Shock*. New York: Random House, 1970. 505 pp.

been anathema 20 years ago. Is there any reason to believe change stops now? What, ultimately, will physicians' assistants do? It was suggested earlier that health educators might be paid as legitimate parts of the health care system. This paragraph began with the prophecy that counselors would be more diverse, and this probably will constitute the largest need and command the least agreement as to what constitutes competence. With these conditions, health care is unlikely to be clearly better. It will be more worrisome for those concerned with high, clearly enforced standards . . . and perhaps seem worse. It predictably will be different.

A CONSERVATIVE FUTURE. But is it the only possible future? Certainly not. Unlikely as it seems at the moment, the culture, in an effort to save itself from feared destruction, might begin to muster majorities that would set certain standards and not tolerate deviations. A cyclic view of history is not necessary, but merely the possibility that the present direction toward extreme tolerance could kindle an opposition that would rise in a crisis. And we would then exchange some freedom for order and security.

SUMMARY. Health is the quality of life being lived. It is a means to the end of fullest total functioning of the whole person. We could be physically healthier if we were not allowed to live as dangerously as we do. We could be mentally healthier (perhaps) if we became less personally competitive. We could be socially healthier if we were forced to a more equitable distribution of what society produces. This leaves us with the haunting prime value question:

> For fullest functioning in all the dimensions of well-being—physical, mental, emotional, social and spiritual—how much of the ingredient freedom is necessary?

**Joint Committee
on Health Problems in Education
of the National Education Association
and the American Medical Association**

Members of the Joint Committee During
Preparation of *Health Education,* Sixth Edition

National Education Association	*American Medical Association*
1968-73 Mary K. Beyrer, Ph.D. Columbus, Ohio	Charles H. McMullen, M.D. (Chairman 72-73) Loudonville, Ohio
1969-74 Miss Nancy Willis (Chairman 73-74) Des Moines, Iowa	Joseph B. Robinson, M.D. Albany, New York
1970-75 Mrs. Margaret B. Kerr Nashville, Tennessee	Marcia F. Curry, M.D. (Chairman 74-75) Denver, Colorado
1971-76 Mrs. Sally R. Williams, R.N. Garden Grove, California	Hilbert P. Jubelt, M.D. Manhattan, Kansas
1972-77 Walter L. Littlejohn, Ed.D. Pine Bluff, Arkansas	Craig D. Ellyson, M.D. Waterloo, Iowa
1973-78 Mr. Harold S. Austin St. Louis, Missouri	Tom W. Robinson, M.D. Newport Beach, California

Joint Committee Liaison Members

John H. Cooper, P.E.D.
NEA Liaison
Washington, D. C.

Wallace Ann Wesley, Hs.D.,
Secretary
AMA Liaison
Chicago, Illinois

Sub-Committee on Revision of *Health Education*

Mrs. Margaret B. Kerr, Chairman
Charles H. McMullen, M.D.
Mary K. Beyrer, Ph.D.
John H. Cooper, P.E.D.
Wallace Ann Wesley, Hs.D.
Elizabeth A. Wilson, Ph.D., Special Consultant
William H. Carlyon, Ph.D., Special Consultant